THE ULTIMATE

Harness the Power of the World's
Healthiest Diet to Live Better, Longer

MEDITERRANEAN DIET

Cookbook

Fair Winds Press
100 Cummings Center, Suite 406L
Beverly, MA 01915

FAIR WINDS

fairwindspress.com • quarryspoon.com

To the memory of my nonna, Angela Magnone Foti, for showing me that food is the foundation upon which our families, communities, cultures, and lives are built

© 2015 Fair Winds Press

First published in the USA in 2015 by
Fair Winds Press, a member of
Quarto Publishing Group USA Inc.
100 Cummings Center
Suite 406-L
Beverly, MA 01915-6101
www.fairwindspress.com
Visit www.QuarrySPOON.com and help us celebrate food and culture one spoonful at a time!

19 18 17 16 15   1 2 3 4 5

ISBN: 978-1-59233-648-7
Digital edition published in 2015
eISBN: 978-1-62788-304-7

Library of Congress Cataloging-in-Publication Data

Riolo, Amy.
 The ultimate Mediterranean diet cookbook : harness the power of the world's healthiest diet to live better, longer / Amy Riolo.
   pages cm
   ISBN 978-1-59233-648-7 (paperback)
 1. Cooking, Mediterranean. 2. Diet--Mediterranean Region. 3. Longevity—Nutritional aspects. I. Title.
 TX725.M35R56 2015
 641.59'1822--dc23

                              2014041235

Cover and book design by Laia Albaladejo
Photography: Glenn Scott Photography; food styling, Natasha Taylor; accent images, Shutterstock.com
Illustration, page 7, Mattie Wells
Printed and bound in China

The information in this book is for educational purposes only. It is not intended to replace the advice of a physician or medical practitioner. Please see your health care provider before beginning any new health program.

Contents

Introduction: Welcome to the Mediterranean Diet

> "Let food be thy medicine, and medicine thy food"—*Hippocrates*

My personal relationship with Mediterranean cuisine did not begin with a so-called diet. It began in the kitchens and at the tables of my grandmothers. With them, I learned that food was not just something to fill our stomachs, but a powerful tool that affected our moods, daily lives, holidays, and wellbeing. Our food provided our family with a sense of tradition and an important cultural rite that connected us with our ancestors and our relatives overseas. To my grandmothers, food was also medicine, and they had an edible remedy for almost every ailment.

Somewhere along the line, however, things changed. As our family became busier and people began relocating for work, many of our traditional foodways were lost. Eating in restaurants and taking medicine began to replace homemade food and natural remedies.

In the United States, the majority of my family members suffer from heart disease, diabetes, hypertension, and high cholesterol. It was a fact of life that I believed to be genetic until I had the opportunity to visit relatives in my ancestral homeland in Calabria, Italy. I was struck by how much healthier they were than our American family. When I asked the Italian relatives about their health, they had, thankfully, no major problems to report. We shared the same genes, the same looks, character traits, and sometimes even the same names, but those who grew up in Italy were decidedly healthier. It was at that moment that I became a fan of the Mediterranean diet and lifestyle.

I ended up returning to Italy not long after that trip and living there for a year. I wanted to truly immerse myself in the culture and reap the benefits of its healthful lifestyle. I also wanted to be able to translate the living traditions into simple acts that anyone, anywhere could incorporate into their lifestyle to achieve optimal health. Years later I had the opportunity to live in and visit other Mediterranean countries, and my research continued. I began searching for commonalities that could benefit people everywhere.

I learned that three factors hold true throughout the Mediterranean region:

- Food is treated as medicine.
- Moderation is key.
- An active physical and social lifestyle is mandatory.

Since these elements have been practiced since antiquity in the twenty-seven countries in the region—countries as diverse as France, Israel, Egypt, and Morocco—they are second nature to the people living there. My mission with *The Ultimate Mediterranean Diet Cookbook* is to illustrate the easiness, effectiveness, and deliciousness of the Mediterranean diet in the most comprehensive, easy to implement, and fun manner possible.

I purposely chose the recipes in this cookbook because of their taste, authenticity, and nutritional value. Not only are most of them low in fat, cholesterol, and sodium, they are also packed with vitamins, minerals, and healthful properties that our bodies crave. The recipes are organized in the same format as the Mediterranean Diet Pyramid, (opposite), offering the most varieties of foods that we should eat the most of, and the least of foods we should limit. Each recipe contains a Mediterranean Tradition to enhance the daily living aspects of the eating plan, and meal plans and serving suggestions are noted, Mediterranean style.

I personally love the Mediterranean diet because it offers great-tasting food with rich traditions attached to them. Just like a multigenerational family sitting at an open air table, the Mediterranean diet pleases all ages and palates. I hope that this book inspires more shared memories at the table, as well as happiness and health to everyone who reads it!

Enjoy with pleasure and health,

—Amy Riolo

The Mediterranean Diet Pyramid

MEATS AND SWEETS
Less often

DRINK WATER

POULTRY, EGGS, CHEESE, AND YOGURT
Moderate portions, daily to weekly

FISH AND SEAFOOD
Often—at least two times per week

WINE
In moderation

FRUITS, VEGETABLES, GRAINS (MOSTLY WHOLE), OLIVE OIL, BEANS, NUTS, LEGUMES AND SEEDS, HERBS, AND SPICES
Base every meal on these foods.

BE PHYSICALLY ACTIVE
Enjoy meals with others

The Healthiest Diet in the World: Benefits of the Mediterranean Diet

> "Sit at dinner tables as long as you can, and converse to your heart's desire, for these are the bonus times of your lives."
> —Al-Hasan bin Abi Talib (grandson of the Prophet Muhammad)

The Mediterranean diet is known as the healthiest in the world because it is not truly a diet, but rather a lifestyle that prescribes a lot of what we should eat, and a little of what we shouldn't, along with shared physical and social activities. Oldways, a nonprofit food and nutrition education organization that features the Mediterranean Diet Pyramid (page 7), refers to the Mediterranean diet as "the gold standard eating pattern that promotes lifelong good health."

The base of the Pyramid shows the importance Mediterranean cultures place on enjoying meals with others and being physically active. Regardless of religion, ethnicity, or language, the people of the Mediterranean region share a common desire to spend time eating and socializing with friends. In the Muslim countries of the Mediterranean region, there are even prophetic sayings encouraging believers to choose who they eat with before they decide what to eat.

The Mediterranean diet, then, is a modern eating plan based on the traditional diet and lifestyle of the countries bordering the Mediterranean Sea. Best of all, while many of the recipes, ingredients, and traditions celebrated in the Mediterranean diet have been around for centuries, they are easily adaptable into today's busy lifestyle and suitable for modern palates. There are no fads, special "diet" foods, or modern technology needed to achieve successful results. There are no formulas, exchanges, or point systems to master. Best of all, you don't need a nutrition label to determine what fits into the lifestyle. Cent ered on healthful, whole foods eaten in moderation, sticking to the Mediterranean diet becomes second nature.

One glance at the Mediterranean Diet Pyramid reveals the majority of items that should be eaten or practiced at the wider, bottom portion of the triangle. The items that should be eaten sparingly appear at the top. All you need to do to successfully follow the Mediterranean diet is switch your mentality to traditional means of preparing and eating natural, whole foods, getting regular physical activity, and making a commitment to prepare and eat foods in community whenever possible.

The Science Behind the Diet

Intrigued by the number of elderly people living with lower rates of illness and disease in the region, scientists and doctors around the world have been researching the Mediterranean diet for more than half a century. Today, large well-designed studies and clinical trials are demonstrating its effects. Following the diet has thus far been linked to:

- preventing heart attacks and strokes
- improved mental capacity
- preventing and reversing diabetes
- reversing the symptoms and reducing the incidence of Parkinson's and Alzheimer's
- longevity
- reduced inflammation
- reduced risk of death from heart disease and cancer
- preventing cancer and inhibiting tumor growth

One impressive study of 7,447 people reported in 2013 in the *New England Journal of Medicine* found that high-risk heart disease subjects could prevent 30 percent of heart attacks, strokes, and deaths from heart disease by switching to a Mediterranean diet. The results were so dramatic that the study was concluded early because the researchers felt that continuing to test control groups following other diets would be unethical when they had already determined the efficacy of the diet.

Another study published in the *Annals of Internal Medicine* tracked the diets and lifestyles of more than 10,000 women in their fifties for fifteen years. The results showed that 40 percent of those who followed the Mediterranean diet were more likely to live past the age of seventy without chronic diseases, memory loss,

or physical problems. They also suffered fewer strokes and were less likely to die than the control group who simply followed a low-fat diet.

It is worth noting that low-fat and Mediterranean diets have different philosophies. Low-fat diets focus on what people should not eat (namely, fat), whereas the notion of deprivation does not fit with the tenets of the Mediterranean diet. So, while following a generally low-fat diet may cut risks associated with higher fat intakes, you will not reap the same rewards that the Mediterranean diet offers.

Many doctors are recommending the Mediterranean diet to combat chronic inflammation, which is an underlying cause or factor in many illnesses, from allergies and arthritis to autoimmune diseases and even cancer. According to Norton Fishman, M.D., F.A.C.P., C.N.S., Medical Director of Optimal Health Physicians in Rockville, MD, it is "key in helping patients with chronic, persistent infections such as Lyme disease. Many of the people suffering from these types of infections develop insulin resistance and gluten sensitivies. The healthful fats and lack of processed grains and sugar associated with a Mediterranean diet are the perfect eating plan."

To prove that the Mediterranean diet can reduce inflammation and impact diabetes, Spanish researchers studied 3,541 Spaniards between the ages of fifty-five and eighty who had three or more risk factors for diabetes. After four years, 87 percent of the high-risk subjects following a Mediterranean diet were able to prevent the onset of diabetes.

The combination of a lifetime of enjoyable meals that taste great and just happen to be good for you is almost too good to be true! One of the most attractive attributes of the diet is that, in essence, it doesn't ask us to give up anything or deprive ourselves: It's a simple strategy that requires exercise, consuming the majority of calories from foods that are good for you, and reserving those that aren't for special occasions.

"In 2008, I was personally and professionally burned out. I realized that I needed to rediscover the importance of a healthy lifestyle through nutrition, physical activity, and mindful living. The work of Daniel Buettner and others, who identified Blue Zones where people live better with greater longevity, also put me in touch with both the cultural and research support that I needed to get back to my Mediterranean heritage. The principles of the Mediterranean diet and lifestyle were so profound for me that they became the cornerstone of a six-week program I designed, the Roadmap to Wellness. These dietary principles have been incorporated into the lifestyles of those who have been most successful in our programs. Food choices based in the Mediterranean diet are about enhancing enjoyment of life through healthy choices."

—John R. Principe, M.D. creator and founder of WellBeingMD, LTD

It's a Lifestyle

It might come as a surprise to many that the base of the Mediterranean Diet Pyramid is not a food group at all, but rather behaviors such as physical activity and social interaction. At its core, the Mediterranean diet is not a diet in the conventional sense of the word. It is a lifestyle that should be enjoyed with both pleasure and health in mind. When people sit down at a table in Egypt, the phrase *bilhanna wi shefa* or "with pleasure and health" is uttered much in the same way that *bon appetit* is in many places. I fell in love with this phrase the first time I heard it; food *should* be about equal parts health and enjoyment.

Physical Activity

The Mediterranean's philosophy of approaching life with an equal measure of pleasure and health leads to a more balanced and happy existence. To the majority of people living in modern urban areas, physical activity means heading off to a gym to work off calories on machines after an entire day's worth of sitting at their desks, in their cars, or on their couches.

In the Mediterranean region, however, it's another story. Daily life is set up to naturally require more activity and calorie expenditure. Urban and commercial areas are built in historic centers that preceded the invention of cars. Driving and parking in them is difficult, which necessitates a greater deal of walking. Electrical capacity is also often lower in many areas, making it difficult to operate many appliances simultaneously. Outside of hotels, few people have clothes dryers, even in urban areas. Simple tasks such as hanging clothes out to dry and ironing them, shopping, and cooking require greater effort and expenditure of calories.

In order to enjoy optimal health and reap the rewards of the Mediterranean diet, followers need to integrate pleasurable forms of activity into their daily lives.

Camaraderie

Every country and culture around the Mediterranean has its own way of encouraging people to eat together, and family life is valued greatly. Throughout the region's history, eating alone was frowned upon. Only unworthy bachelors or scorned people who didn't have family would eat by themselves. While attitudes have changed in modern times, most people in the Mediterranean find it unpleasant to eat alone. Fortunately, in many places, work and school schedules revolve around mealtimes. When they do not, families change their schedules in order to be able to eat together at least for one meal per day.

Residents on the Mediterranean island of Sardinia are ten times more likely to live past 100 than people in the United States. Researchers who studied this remarkable longevity found that daily communal (family style) eating was commonplace and attributed it to the overall wellbeing of residents. The researchers concluded that there is something extremely satisfying and comforting about knowing that, no matter how difficult life gets, at lunchtime you will be surrounded by loved ones. This adds a deep sense of psychological security, which, in turn, has a positive effect on health and happiness.

> ### Ground Rules for Rewarding Family Meals
>
> 1. No television or electronics
> 2. No off-limits or unpleasant topics
> 3. Dress for the meal.
> 4. Set as attractive a table as possible.
> 5. Discuss pleasant topics and good news.

Throughout the region, food is viewed as a way to express love, thanks, appreciation, and respect. It may be used as a gift, as a way to settle a debt, or as a traditional medicine. In southern European countries such as Spain, Italy, Greece, and France, great pride is taken in giving a guest or a loved one a handmade food item; if it was grown on the giver's own land, it is even more special. What comes from the hands is an extension of self—and is healthier than what can be bought at the store. When my relatives came to visit me in the United States from Calabria, Italy, they brought finely ground chile pepper, cheese, olives, and cured meats, all of which were produced on the family's farm.

As I share these thoughts and reflections, I realize that, in our busy day-to-day existence, much of what I am describing sounds like a Utopian fantasy. While most Americans will find re-creating this type of lifestyle unrealistic, I propose simple ways to implement it:

- Vow to live each day with both pleasure and health in mind.
- Find easy, enjoyable ways to get more exercise, such as gardening or walking with a friend.
- Begin incorporating new and varied plant-based foods into your diet.
- Identify simple, make-ahead dishes and snacks to work into your schedule.
- If it is not already a custom, make plans to eat, exercise, and socialize with friends, family, and co-workers as often as possible.
- Treat food, family, and friends as if they are the most important part of your life.

Plant-Based Foods: The Foundation of the Mediterranean Diet

> "I recommend the Mediterranean diet to patients because it is based predominantly on plant-based foods, which offer nutritional benefits and protein, yet no cholesterol. Many people are surprised to learn that delicious ingredients like avocados and almonds are cholesterol free."
> —*Martha Kern, M.D. (internist)*

Medical doctors and supporters of the Mediterranean diet believe that, for optimal health, a variety of plant foods should make up the majority of our meals. Residents of Greece consume an average of six or more servings of fruits and vegetables a day, which is nothing unique in the Mediterranean region, where a cornucopia of fresh, ripe produce is inexpensive, delicious, and readily available.

In countries outside the Mediterranean, the challenges of procuring local, organic produce on a daily basis can be overcome by planning ahead and shopping smartly. Maintain a list of seasonal produce available in your area, and you can reap the rewards of incorporating more of these nutritional powerhouses into your diet.

This chapter covers the largest, food-centric level of the Mediterranean Diet Pyramid, which includes whole grains, fruits, vegetables, legumes and nuts, and olive oil.

WHOLE GRAINS

Grains are the backbone of the Mediterranean diet. French baguettes, Italian pastas, Egyptian pita bread, Turkish rice pilafs, and Libyan couscous all hold a special place in my heart and on the tables in their respective countries. Many varieties of grain, such as barley, buckwheat, farro, spelt, wheat, and wheat berries have been enjoyed in the Mediterranean region for millennia. Others, such as rice and corn, were introduced after the discovery of the New World. Quinoa, a seed of South American origin, is the newest import, and became fashionable in the last decade due to its popularity in the United States. And, even though potatoes are not technically grains, I have chosen to include them in this section because, like grains, they contain significant amounts of carbohydrates and are viewed culturally as a grain alternative.

Grains were once an important currency that entire empires, including ancient Egypt, were built on. So integral were grains and the food they produced that the ancient Egyptian word for bread, *aish*, actually means life. In ancient Egypt, Greece, and Italy, special breads were baked to honor the pharaohs and the gods. Later, these culinary offerings were woven into Christian traditions, and were baked for holidays and to honor the saints. Many Judeo-Islamic traditions involved grains as well.

Throughout Mediterranean history, finely milled flours became associated with the upper classes and coarser grains with poorer communities. Average people couldn't afford the finely milled flour that is used in making today's pasta. As a result, many types of whole grains and grasses were combined to make traditional pastas. But, as we now know, excessive milling strips grains of their nutritional benefits. Therefore, choosing organic, heirloom, whole grains whenever possible is a great way to adhere to the Mediterranean diet, reap its health benefits, and eat what is culturally appropriate. There is no need to eschew wheat or grain completely because of recent headlines or diet fads.

There is a strong prejudice against wheat–based foods in some countries that the Mediterranean region does not suffer from. For starters, most of the wheat grown in the Mediterranean is not genetically modified. It is the same type of wheat that has been grown since antiquity; it offers more nutrients and is more easily digested by the body. (For those who suffer from gluten intolerance, I've included a gluten-free alternative in recipes containing it.)

Nutritional Benefits

According to the Cleveland Clinic, a study involving nearly two million people found that eating 3¼ ounces (100 g) of high-fiber whole grains per day reduced the risk of colorectal cancer, the second leading cancer killer in the United States, by 20 percent. Obesity, diabetes, and heart disease were also reduced when patients ate good sources of soluble fiber, which helps you to feel fuller longer, and reduces cholesterol. Whole grains also contain glutamic acid, which is believed to help lower blood pressure.

The caloric density of whole grains is low, which means that you can eat more of them and feel satisfied while taking in small amounts of calories. Since dietary and saturated fat intake also play a role in the development of heart disease, it is important to keep them to a minimum in addition to consuming whole grains in order to achieve their maximum benefits. Fortunately, the Mediterranean diet naturally allows for this.

One Italian grain to look for is *grano duro,* a hard winter wheat flour that takes center stage in pasta making. Semolina is made from *grano duro* flour. The semolina itself is known as the heart of wheat, whereas semolina flour is often made from mixing the leftover bran and germ layers of the wheat. As the second most commonly used wheat in the world, durum wheat, or *Triticum Durum,* as it is known in Latin, offers a higher amount of protein (16 percent), B vitamins, folic acid, and phosphorus than other varieties, and it contains no cholesterol. It also contains six of nine essential amino acids, making it an excellent choice for vegetarians.

Senatore Capelli wheat is high in vitamins, minerals, lipids, and protein. It has also been found to be safe for many people with gluten intolerances—though check with your health care practitioner first. Many modern *pastifici,* or pasta makers, have been offering traditionally made pastas using this type of flour, and it is becoming very fashionable among home consumers and restaurants.

If whole grains are new for you, be aware that adding fiber to your diet can add bulk to stool; it is therefore important to drink increased amounts of water as you add more fiber. When incorporating new or additional whole grains into the diet, aim for one additional serving per week.

Borlotti Bean Soup with Basil/
Zuppa di borlotti e basilico

In Italy, a *minestra* is a thick soup made from a multitude of ingredients, which explains why there are so many ingredients in this recipe. Adding the suffix -*one* on the end means that it is a large or big *minestra*. To make this dish vegetarian, substitute vegetable stock for the chicken stock.

1 tablespoon (15 ml) extra-virgin olive oil

1 medium yellow onion, finely chopped

2 carrots, finely chopped

1 rib celery, finely chopped

¼ cup (15 g) flat-leaf parsley, chopped

6 cloves garlic, chopped

3 cups (210 g) shredded cabbage

1 Yukon gold potato, peeled and chopped into bite-size pieces

8 cups (2 L) reduced-sodium Chicken Stock (see page 183)

2 zucchini, peeled and chopped into bite-size pieces

2 large tomatoes, chopped

½ pound (225 g) string beans, chopped into bite-size pieces

2 cups (390 g) cooked borlotti (cranberry) beans

Unrefined sea salt or salt

Freshly ground pepper

½ cup (60 g) freshly grated Pecorino Romano cheese

Yield: 8 servings

Heat the olive oil in a large stockpot over medium heat. Add the onion, carrot, and celery, and stir. Sauté for 3 to 5 minutes or until tender. Add the parsley and garlic, and cook for 1 minute longer.

Stir in the cabbage and potato. Pour in the chicken stock, increase heat to high, and bring to a boil. Add the zucchini, tomatoes, string beans, borlotti beans, salt, and pepper. Cover, lower heat, and allow to simmer for 40 minutes to 1 hour, or until vegetables are tender.

Taste, and adjust seasonings, if necessary. Use a ladle to transfer half of the soup to a blender. Remove the spout on the lid and cover with a folded kitchen towel. Purée until smooth, and return to stockpot. Stir to blend. Serve hot, topped with Pecorino Romano cheese.

Mediterranean Tradition

Minestre are the ultimate in cupboard cooking. In my ancestral homeland of Calabria, Italy, a thick *minestra* called *mille cosedde* or "a thousand things" is made by cleaning out the cupboards on New Year's Eve. Small pasta, lentils (which symbolize good fortune), at least three different kinds of beans, vegetables, and stock are all added to the pot. The result is a unique, delicious, and extremely economical soup that varies from year to year. Try using this recipe as a guideline and substituting the ingredients you have on hand to come up with your own version.

Whole-Wheat Pita Bread/*Aish Baladi*

Whole-wheat pita bread dates back to the twentieth century BCE in ancient Egypt. Under Roman rule, wheat flour from Egypt and North Africa was exported throughout the Roman Empire, and similar recipes spread throughout the Mediterranean. The Roman philosopher Apicius even mentioned the "bread from Alexandria" in his cookbook *De Re Coquinaria*.

1⅛ cups (265 ml) warm water

1 tablespoon (12 g) active dry yeast

½ tablespoon (9 g) unrefined sea salt or salt

2 cups (250 g) whole-wheat flour (see Gluten-Free Alternative)

1½ cups (188 g) unbleached, all-purpose flour (see Gluten-Free Alternative)

1 tablespoon (15 ml) extra-virgin olive oil

Yield: 6 pitas

Pour the water into a large bowl. Add the yeast and stir until dissolved. Add the salt, and gradually incorporate the flours to form a dough.

Turn the dough out onto a lightly floured work surface and knead for 10 minutes, until smooth and elastic. Or place in the bowl of an electric mixer fitted with a hook attachment and knead on medium speed for 2 minutes.

Pour the oil into a bowl and place dough inside the bowl, turning to coat. Cover with oiled plastic and a kitchen towel and let rise until doubled in bulk (1½ to 2 hours).

When the dough has risen, punch down gently. Divide the dough into six equal portions and shape into balls. Place on a lightly floured surface and cover with a dry kitchen towel. Let rest for 15 minutes.

Preheat the oven to 475°F (240°C). Place a baking stone or sheet in lowest section of oven. Roll out each dough circle to form a 6-inch (15 cm) circle. Place three circles on the preheated baking sheet and bake for about 12 minutes (until they are puffed up and begin to turn color). Refrain from opening the oven during the first 4 minutes of cooking. Remove with a metal spatula or pizza peel and place in a bread basket or on a serving platter. Repeat with the remaining dough circles until all are baked.

Gluten-Free Alternative:
Replace the flours in this recipe with a combination of 1½ cups (237 g) brown rice flour, 1 cup (125 g) tapioca flour, 1 cup (136 g) sorghum flour, and 2 teaspoons xanthan gum.

Mediterranean Tradition
Fresh breads go stale quickly because they lack the preservatives that give commercial breads a longer shelf life. For that reason, savvy cooks in the region have been utilizing day-old breads in countless ways for millennia. Try cutting this day-old bread into cubes, drizzling it with olive oil, and a sprinkling with *za'atar* spice or Pecorino Romano cheese. Place on a baking sheet and toast in a 400°F (200°C) oven until golden. The croutons are a perfect addition to salads, soups, stews, and casseroles.

Mediterranean-Style Corn Bread/
Pane di mais con mozzarella e pomodori secchi

Even though corn is native to the Americas, its popularity in the Mediterranean region is so widespread that you would think it originated there. This Italian-inspired version is an updated interpretation of traditional recipes from the northern Italian regions of Veneto, Lombardia, and Fruili. Introduced by the Ottomans in the 900s, corn flour was called *grano turco,* or "Turkish grains" in Italian, and became extremely popular with the Jewish community in Venice. Soon thereafter, it became a poor man's staple throughout Italy.

2 teaspoons extra-virgin olive oil, divided

2½ cups (305 g) stone ground 100% whole-grain, medium-grind cornmeal

½ tablespoon (9 g) unrefined sea salt or salt

2 teaspoons baking powder

1 teaspoon sugar

2 cups (475 ml) boiling water

¼ cup (14 g) chopped sun-dried tomatoes

4 ounces (115 g) fresh mozzarella cheese, shredded by hand into large pieces

Yield: 12 servings

Preheat the oven to 350°F (180°C).

Grease an 8-inch (20 cm) round cake pan with 1 teaspoon olive oil.

Combine the cornmeal, salt, remaining 1 teaspoon olive oil, baking powder, and sugar in a large bowl. Add the boiling water and stir to mix until all of the water is incorporated in the mixture.

Stir in the sun-dried tomatoes and mozzarella. Pour the cornmeal mixture into the prepared pan. Wet your hands and press down to smooth the top.

Bake for 10 minutes and then cover the pan with aluminum foil and bake for 20 to 30 minutes, or until golden and firm on top. Allow to cool slightly and serve warm, or allow to cool and wrap in plastic wrap.

Mediterranean Tradition
While many Americans find the words *healthful bread* to be an oxymoron, this isn't the case in the Mediterranean region. There, fresh breads made with high-quality grains are enjoyed daily and are a backbone to the diet. Simple, quick breads such as this one can be whipped up in minutes and provide a heartier alternative to store-bought varieties.

Whole-Wheat Pizza/*Pizza Integrale*

Pizza dough dates back to antiquity and has roots in Egypt, Greece, and Rome. Modern pizza (with a tomato topping) was first served in eighteenth-century Naples, Italy, using tomatoes, which were recently imported from the New World, and traditional buffalo-milk mozzarella. Simple grilled or panfried chicken, veal, beef, or seafood are natural accompaniments. If you are using fresh tomatoes, skin them and put them through a food mill to remove the seeds. Canned or boxed strained tomatoes can be found in gourmet and import stores and are great time savers. This sauce will keep in the refrigerator for up to 1 week or in the freezer for a few months.

For the Dough:

1 package (¼ ounce, or 7 g) active dry yeast

½ cup (120 ml) lukewarm water

1½ cups (188 g) whole-wheat flour, plus extra for work surface (see Gluten-Free Alternative)

1 teaspoon kosher salt

1 tablespoon (15 ml) extra-virgin olive oil, plus extra for bowl

For the Sauce:

1 tablespoon (15 ml) extra-virgin olive oil

1 large clove garlic, minced

¾ pound (340 g) strained (seeded and skinned) tomatoes, such as Pomi brand

Unrefined sea salt or salt, to taste

Freshly ground pepper, to taste

1 tablespoon (2.5 g) finely chopped fresh basil, oregano, or parsley

2 tablespoons (18 g) cornmeal or semolina

10 ounces (288 g) fresh mozzarella cheese, grated

Grated Parmigiano-Reggiano or Pecorino Romano cheese

Yield: 1 pizza

To make the dough: Place the yeast in a small bowl and stir in the water. Set aside. Put the flour into a large bowl and add the yeast to the center. Add the salt and olive oil, and stir to combine until it forms a dense dough that will be slightly sticky. If the dough does not come together, add more water, a tablespoon (15 ml) at a time.

Dust a work surface lightly with flour. Knead the dough energetically for 5 to 10 minutes, or until it is smooth and supple. Shape the dough into a ball and place it in a lightly oiled bowl. Cover with oiled plastic and a clean kitchen cloth. Allow to rise for 1½ to 2 hours, or until doubled in size. In the meantime, make the sauce.

To make the sauce: Heat the oil in a medium saucepan over medium heat. Add garlic and reduce heat to low.

When the garlic begins to release its aroma (before it turns color), add the tomatoes. Stir and allow the mixture to come to a boil. Add salt, pepper, and fresh herbs, stir and cover. Reduce heat to low and simmer for 20 to 30 minutes. Allow to cool.

Finishing the pizza: When the dough has finished rising, preheat the oven to 500°F to 550°F (250°C to 288°C). Punch the dough down and let it rest 5 minutes. Use a rolling pin to roll it out into a 10- to 12-inch (26 to 30 cm) diameter circle. Transfer to a pizza stone or peel dusted with cornmeal or semolina.

Cover the dough with a thin layer of sauce, mozzarella, and a sprinkling of Pecorino or Parmigiano cheese. Fold the edges of the crust in and brush lightly with extra olive oil. Bake on the second-to-lowest rack for 10 to 15 minutes or until golden and bubbly. Remove from the oven and allow to stand 5 minutes. Cut and serve.

Gluten-Free Alternative:

Substitute whole-wheat flour with ¾ cup (94 g) tapioca flour, ½ cup (79 g) white rice flour, ¼ cup (23 g) chickpea flour, ¼ cup (34 g) sorghum flour, and 1 teaspoon xanthan gum.

Mediterranean Tradition

Mediterranean cooks are always thinking ahead! Keep in mind that you can double the recipes for pizza dough and sauce and freeze them so that you will have them ready for another occasion.

Whole-Wheat and Grape Focaccia/*Schiacciata all'uva*

Schiacciata, the name of this delicious bread in Italian, is derived from the verb *schiacciare,* which means "flattened out" and that's exactly what happens when freshly harvested grapes are pressed into it. Traditionally made at grape harvest time in Tuscany, this recipe originated with the Etruscans and was baked in the ashes of an open hearth.

1½ cups (425 ml) warm water

½ cup (120 ml) Vin Santo (Italian dessert wine)

1 package (¼ ounce, or 7 g) active dry yeast

½ cup (118 ml) extra-virgin olive oil, divided, plus extra for greasing pan

3 cups (375 g) whole-wheat flour (see Gluten-Free Alternative)

1 cup (125 g) unbleached, all-purpose flour (see Gluten-Free Alternative)

1 teaspoon unrefined sea salt or salt

2 cups (300 g) seedless red grapes, cut in half lengthwise

Yield: 8 to 10 servings

Pour the water and Vin Santo in the bowl of a standing mixer. Sprinkle the yeast over the top, and mix using the paddle attachment until combined. Let set for 5 minutes. Pour in ¼ cup (60 ml) of olive oil. Add the whole-wheat flour and mix on low speed. Slowly add in the all-purpose flour and salt, and mix until well combined.

Switch to the dough hook attachment and knead the dough on medium speed for 5 minutes. Cover the bowl with oiled plastic wrap and allow to rest at room temperature until doubled in size, about 1 hour (see note).

Oil a 13 x 17-inch (33 x 43 cm) rimmed baking sheet. Turn the dough from the bowl onto the baking sheet. Stretch the dough out and press down until it covers the surface of the pan in an even layer.

Using all the fingers of your hands, press down to make dimples in the surface of the focaccia. Cover with oiled plastic wrap and allow to rest for 30 minutes, or until the dough has doubled in size again.

Preheat the oven to 425°F (220°C).

Before baking, brush the surface of the focaccia with the remaining ¼ cup (60 ml) of olive oil. Scatter the grapes, cut side down over the top and press them down slightly. Bake for 30 to 35 minutes, or until the focaccia turns a nice golden brown and is cooked through. Remove from the oven and allow to cool slightly. Cut and serve immediately. Leftover, cooled pieces can be wrapped in plastic wrap and frozen for up to 1 month.

Gluten-Free Alternative:
Substitute the flour in this recipe with 1½ cups (188 g) tapioca flour, 1⅓ cups (181 g) sorghum flour, ⅔ cup (129 g) potato starch, ½ cup (79 g) sweet rice flour, and 1 teaspoon xanthan gum.

Note: If you would like to make this dough in the morning to eat in the evening, cover the bowl with plastic wrap and a clean kitchen towel and place in the refrigerator. In 12 hours, you will have the same results as if it sat at room temperature for 1 hour.

Mediterranean Tradition
Using fresh fruit in as many ways possible is something that chefs and home cooks in the Mediterranean region take great pride in. Challenge yourself to go outside of your culinary comfort zone when garden-fresh fruits are readily available—you'll be sure to discover new favorites and increase your plant–based food intake.

Bulgur Pilaf with Chestnuts/*Kestaneli Bulgur Pilavi*

This delicious yet simple and healthful pilaf hails from the town of Bursa, Turkey. The recipe is adapted from *The Turkish Cookbook: Regional Recipes and Stories* by Nur Ilkin and Sheilah Kaufman, who write, "Chestnuts are full of fiber and low in fat. They are used in a wide variety of Marmara [region in Turkey] dishes as a paste, puréed, or roasted."

4 tablespoons (59 ml) extra-virgin olive oil

3 medium onions, finely chopped

2 cups (280 g) coarse bulgur (see Gluten-Free Alternative)

4 cups (940 ml) Chicken Stock (page 183)

2 tablespoons (18 g) dried sultanas or dried currants, soaked in water to cover for 1 hour

1 teaspoon allspice

1 teaspoon cumin

Unrefined sea salt or salt, to taste

1 package (5.28 ounces, or 150 g) roasted, shelled chestnuts

Yield: 6 to 8 servings

In a medium-size pan, heat the olive oil and sauté the onions for 5 to 6 minutes, until softened. Add the coarse bulgur and chicken stock, mix well, and bring to a boil. Stir in the sultanas or currants, allspice, cumin, salt, and chestnuts. Reduce heat to a simmer, cover, and cook until all the liquid has been absorbed and holes start to form on the surface, 15 to 20 minutes.

Remove from the heat, remove lid, place a double layer of paper towel over the bulgur, cover, and let sit for 10 to 15 minutes. Mix well and serve with any main course.

Gluten-Free Alternative:
Substitute 2 cups (346 g) quinoa, 1⅓ cups (266 g) millet, or 2 cups (370 g) extra-long-grain white rice for bulgur.

Mediterranean Tradition
Chestnuts contain high amounts of vitamin B, a fat soluble vitamin that helps promote healthy skin and improve brain function. They also break down protein, carbohydrates, and fats for energy. Try eating roasted chestnuts with leafy greens and lean proteins for a vitamin B–packed meal.

Lebanese Pumpkin Kibbeh/*Kibbeh Laqteen*

The Orthodox Christian communities of the Mediterranean region observe religious fasts during which all dairy, seafood, meat, and poultry are off limits for long periods of time. In order to make up for the fat, flavor, and heartiness in the foods they must abstain from, the Lebanese, Syrians, Egyptians, Greeks, and others who observe the Eastern Orthodox calendar have come up with extremely flavorful and unique vegan dishes over the centuries. This one replaces the traditional kibbeh—a dish especially popular in Lebanon that combines bulgur wheat with ground meat, nuts, herbs, and spices in dozens of ingenious and mouthwatering ways. The kibbeh are fried in torpedo-shaped croquettes or layered in pans and baked in the oven. During the Lenten period, they are filled with vegetables, as in this pumpkin version.

1½ cups (210 g) of fine bulgur #1 (see Gluten-Free Alternative)

4 tablespoons (60 ml) extra-virgin olive oil, divided

2 large onions, chopped

1 pound (455 g) fresh spinach, cleaned and trimmed

2 cups (480 g) cooked chickpeas (see page 182)

3 tablespoons (23 g) sumac

1 teaspoon unrefined sea salt or salt

¼ teaspoon ground white pepper

2 pounds (910 g) chunked cooked pumpkin

1 cup (50 g) Fresh Bread Crumbs (see page 182)

2 teaspoons Aleppo pepper or good-quality paprika

1 teaspoon cumin

1 teaspoon dried coriander

1 teaspoon ground cinnamon

1 teaspoon allspice

⅓ cup (45 g) pine nuts, toasted

Yield: 6 to 8 servings

Rinse the bulgur in a fine mesh colander. Place in a medium bowl and cover with water, until it fluffs up and is soft, 5 to 10 minutes. Drain, if necessary, and set aside.

Heat 2 tablespoons (30 ml) of olive oil in a large saucepan over medium heat. Add the onions and sauté, stirring occasionally, 3 to 5 minutes, or until golden. Add the spinach and stir until wilted. Remove from the heat and stir in the chickpeas. Stir in the sumac, salt, and white pepper.

Preheat the oven to 350°F (180°C). Combine the bulgur with the pumpkin in a large bowl, and stir in bread crumbs. Add in the Aleppo pepper or paprika, cumin, dried coriander, cinnamon, and allspice. Taste and adjust salt if necessary.

Grease a 10-inch (26 cm) round cake pan with 2-inch (5 cm) side and press half of the bulgur along the bottom. Place the spinach–onion filling mixture in an even layer across the top. Add the remainder of the bulgur across the top. Use a piece of plastic wrap to help spread the mixture.

Score the surface of the kibbeh in a diagonal pattern. Scatter pine nuts over the top and press down gently. Drizzle remaining 2 tablespoons (30 ml) of olive oil over the top and bake for 30 to 40 minutes, or until golden.

Gluten-Free Alternative:
Substitute 3 cups (555 g) cooked quinoa for the bulgur in this recipe. Press 1½ cups (277 g) along the bottom of the pan, use the filling, and press remaining quinoa over the top.

Mediterranean Tradition
If you're buying bulgur for the first time to make this recipe, you may want to buy extra. It's ready in just minutes after being soaked in water at room temperature and can be used as the base for tabbouleh salad, stirred into soups, tossed with vegetables for a quick pilaf, or combined with milk, fruit, and nuts for a delicious cereal in the morning. Look for sumac in Mediterranean markets.

Herb and Rice-Stuffed Grape Leaves/*Warag Aghnib*

Stuffed grape leaves are synonymous with home, family, and holidays in most parts of the Mediterranean. Enjoyed everywhere from Morocco and across North Africa to Greece, the eastern Mediterranean and Levant, and the Arabian Peninsula, every cook has their own special version, often made with fresh grape leaves. Fresh California grape leaves can be found in some Mediterranean and Middle Eastern markets during grape season, but those sold in glass jars make good substitutes. Soak the jarred variety in boiling water before using to remove the briny taste.

½ pound (225 g) fresh grape vine leaves or 1 jar (8 ounces, or 225 g) preserved vine leaves, drained

1 cup (195 g) medium-grain white rice

⅓ cup (5 g) fresh cilantro, finely chopped

⅓ cup (20 g) fresh parsley, finely chopped

⅓ cup (16 g) fresh dill, finely chopped

⅓ cup (32 g) fresh mint, finely chopped

1 cup (226 g) no-sodium-added canned or boxed, chopped or diced tomatoes, divided

1 medium yellow onion, grated (about ½ cup, or 80 g)

¼ cup (60 ml) extra-virgin olive oil

1 teaspoon kosher salt

1 teaspoon ground coriander

1 teaspoon cumin

Pinch freshly ground black pepper

Pinch chili powder

2 lemons, sliced

1 cup (200 g) Greek yogurt, for serving

Yield: 12 appetizer servings (3 or 4 vine leaves each)

If using preserved vine leaves, place them in a large bowl. Cover with boiling water and let stand for 10 minutes, then drain.

In a medium bowl, mix the rice, cilantro, parsley, dill, mint, ¾ cup (170 g) of the tomatoes, onion, olive oil, salt, coriander, cumin, pepper, and chili powder.

Place 1 leaf on a work surface, vein side up. Cut the excess piece of stem from the bottom of each leaf.

Place 1 tablespoon (15 g) of filling into the middle of each leaf. Shape the filling to resemble the width of a pencil across the width of the leaf.

Roll the leaf up, starting at the bottom. Tuck in the sides of the leaf as you go, making an envelope. Refrain from rolling the leaves too tightly or they will tear as the rice cooks and expands inside. Continue with the remaining leaves.

Place the stuffed vine leaves, seam side down, next to each other in a heavy saucepan. The stuffed leaves should be touching one another and fit into the pan without any spaces.

Repeat a second layer on top, if necessary. Place a plate upside down on top of vine leaves in the saucepan to keep them from rising.

Pour boiling water over the stuffed vine leaves until they are almost, but not completely, covered.

Add the remaining ¼ cup (56 g) tomatoes and additional salt and pepper to taste, if necessary, to the pan.

Cover the saucepan and simmer on low heat until the rice is fully cooked and the leaves are tender, about 1 to 1½ hours. To test the doneness of the stuffed vine leaves, break one in half and taste it. Serve warm or at room temperature with lemon slices and yogurt.

Mediterranean Tradition

This recipe is most fun when it is made in community! The same filling can be used to stuff tomatoes, Cubanelle peppers, baby eggplants, cabbage, and baby zucchini. It is customary to stuff whatever vegetable is in season due to availability, but there are health benefits as well: eating in-season, local produce is actually healthier for us because it provides our bodies with the nutrients that we need during that particular season.

North African Spice-Dusted Sweet Potatoes/ *Batatas Hamras*

Although potatoes where actually introduced into the Mediterranean after the Spaniards brought them back from the New World, they gained popularity in a short time. Along the Mediterranean shores of many North African countries, sweet potatoes are grilled over coals and sold on the street. Couples usually stop by and pick them up during their romantic evening strolls. Therefore, the Arabic term, *Qul Batatas* or "Eating Potatoes" is often synonymous with being in love.

2 sweet potatoes, about ½ pound (225 g) each, scrubbed

2 tablespoons (30 ml) extra-virgin olive oil

1 teaspoon unrefined sea salt or salt

1 tablespoon (6 g) freshly ground pepper

1 teaspoon pure cinnamon

Yield: 4 servings

Preheat the oven to 400°F (200°C). Prick the sweet potatoes with a fork and place in the middle of the oven. Bake for about 1 hour or until soft when pressed.

Halve the sweet potatoes by splitting lengthwise and making crisscross cuts in the flesh. Drizzle olive oil evenly over the flesh of the four halves. Sprinkle the salt, pepper, and cinnamon over each one. Serve hot.

Note: Cinnamon, native to Asia and introduced to Africa by European traders, has been enjoyed in the Mediterranean since antiquity. It has been found to regulate blood sugar levels of people with Type II diabetes. (The study used pure cinnamon, not the common American variety that contains cassia.) Pure cinnamon—sometimes called true cinnamon, Ceylon cinnamon, or Sri Lankan cinnamon—is becoming more readily available in the United States and has a milder, sweeter, flavor. The consumption of sweet potatoes is believed to help balance the glycemic index of diabetics. When paired together, both their taste and nutritional benefits are powerful!

Mediterranean Tradition
You don't have to travel to North Africa to enjoy grilled sweet potatoes! To make your own, simply halve them, brush them with olive oil, and place them over a moderately heated grill, turning occasionally, until soft. Alternately, you can cut them into 1-inch (2.5 cm) cubes, brush them with olive oil and salt, wrap them in foil and place them over a grill. Cook, turning halfway through, for 10 minutes on each side, or until soft.

Potatoes with Kale, Garlic, Olive Oil, and Chile Pepper/
Patate con ravizzone, aglio e peperoncino

This delicious side dish is a nutritional powerhouse! Potatoes contain antioxidants and phytochemicals that strengthen the immune system, lower inflammation, and prevent tumor growth. According to webmd.com, "One cup of chopped kale contains 33 calories and 9% of the daily value of calcium, 206% of vitamin A, 134% of vitamin C, and a whopping 684% of vitamin K."

4 medium Yukon gold potatoes, chopped into bite-size pieces

4 tablespoons (60 ml) extra-virgin olive oil, divided

4 cloves garlic, finely chopped

Crushed red chile pepper

Unrefined sea salt or salt

Freshly ground pepper to taste

½ pound (225 g) fresh kale, rinsed with stems and tough ribs discarded, then roughly chopped

Yield: 4 servings

Preheat the oven to 450°F (230°C).

Place the potatoes on a baking sheet and combine them with 2 tablespoons (30 ml) of oil, garlic, crushed red chile pepper, salt, and pepper, and bake for 15 to 20 minutes, until golden and soft.

In a large bowl, toss the kale with the remaining 2 tablespoons (30 ml) of oil along with salt and pepper to taste. When the potatoes have roasted, remove from the oven and scatter the kale on top of them. Return to the oven and roast for another 10 minutes, or until kale is crisp. Serve hot.

Mediterranean Tradition

Kale is one of the few vegetables that grows well in cooler temperatures. It can be sautéed, added into soups and pasta dishes, eaten raw in salad, or baked. Choose kale that has strong, deeply colored leaves with thick stems. Fresh kale can be wrapped in paper towels and stored, unwashed, in airtight zippered plastic bags for up to five days in the refrigerator.

Spanish Bravas-Style Potatoes/*Papas Bravas*

Bravas potatoes are a Spanish classic. They are prepared differently in various regions in Spain, but are always part of a tapas meal. Tapas, which means "to cover," refers to small plates or appetizers, served hot or cold in Spanish bars where diners are encouraged to socialize and try various foods. Once upon a time in their native Andalusia, sherry drinkers would cover their glasses with pieces of bread or meat in order to keep the flies away—and soon the food became the main event! The word *bravas* means "fierce" and refers to the heat from the hot pepper sauce added to the recipe.

1 large plum tomato, halved and seeded

2 large Russet potatoes, peeled and cut into 1-inch (2.5 cm) cubes

Pure olive oil

2 cloves garlic, finely chopped

1 tablespoon (7 g) smoked paprika

½ cup (115 g) good-quality or homemade mayonnaise

Few dashes hot pepper sauce

1 tablespoon (15 ml) aged sherry vinegar

Unrefined sea salt or salt

Freshly ground black pepper

Flat-leaf parsley leaves

Yield: 4 servings

Preheat the oven to 425°F (220°C). Roast the tomato halves on a baking sheet until soft, 15 to 20 minutes. Remove and cool.

Reduce the oven to 375°F (190°C). Place a baking sheet in the oven.

Fill a medium saucepan three-quarters full with water. Add the potato cubes and a pinch of salt. Bring to a boil, uncovered, over high heat. Reduce heat to medium, and cook until just fork-tender, 5 to 10 minutes. Drain.

Heat 1 tablespoon (15 ml) of oil in a small frying pan over medium heat. Add the garlic and cook until it releases its aroma, about 3 minutes. Add the paprika and cook for 30 seconds. Let cool slightly.

Combine the garlic and oil mixture, mayonnaise, tomato halves, hot pepper sauce, and vinegar in a food processor and process until smooth. Season with salt and pepper, to taste. Set aside.

Heat 2 inches (5 cm) of pure olive oil in a large high-sided, heavy-bottomed skillet until it begins to shimmer, or reaches 300°F (150°C). Carefully lower in half of the potatoes, and cook until golden brown on all sides.

Remove the potatoes to a paper towel–lined plate for a moment to drain the excess oil, and season with salt and pepper. Repeat with the remaining potatoes. Carefully remove the hot baking sheet from the oven, put the potatoes on the pan in an even layer and bake until crisp, about 10 minutes.

Taste, and adjust seasonings if necessary. Transfer to a platter and garnish with a drizzle of the aioli and the parsley leaves. Serve hot.

Mediterranean Tradition
Use the Andalusians as inspiration when planning meals: A few small plates of exquisitely prepared vegetables, nuts, cheeses, and olives make a delicious, nutritiously valuable, and delicious deviation from the standard dinner plate.

Libyan Lamb Couscous/*Couscous bil Lahma Dani*

In North Africa, lamb couscous is about as hard to come by as sand. I've eaten this dish in its many guises, but am partial to the Libyan version. A few years ago, I was invited to the residence of the Ambassador of Libya to the United States for a small, private dinner party. This lamb couscous was the crowning glory of an elegant and refined meal. The combination of tender lamb meat, aromatic spices, perfectly cooked vegetables, and buttery couscous raised the bar on couscous for me, and I haven't found anything that could compare ever since.

3 tablespoons (45 ml) olive oil

2 pounds (910 g) lamb shoulder or leg meat, with bones, cut into 2 to 3-inch (5 to 7.5 cm) pieces

2 medium onions, finely chopped

1 teaspoon ground turmeric

1½ teaspoons unrefined sea salt or salt, divided

½ teaspoon ground black pepper

½ teaspoon cayenne pepper, if desired

2 tablespoons (32 g) tomato paste

2½ cups (570 ml) Chicken Stock (see page 183)

3 carrots, peeled and cut into 3-inch (7.5 cm) cubes

2 medium potatoes, peeled and cut into 3-inch (7.5 cm) cubes

3 medium zucchini, cut into 3-inch (7.5 cm) cubes

1 cup (240 g) cooked chickpeas (see page 182)

2 cups (314 g) couscous (see Gluten-Free Alternative)

2 tablespoons (28 g) butter

Yield: 4 servings

Heat the oil in a large heavy-bottomed saucepan over medium heat. Add the meat and brown on all sides. Add the onions, stir, and sauté until tender, 5 minutes.

Season with turmeric, 1 teaspoon salt, pepper, and cayenne (if using), and stir in the tomato paste. Cook, uncovered for 2 more minutes.

Pour in the stock, cover and simmer for 1½ hours, or until the meat is tender.

Add the carrots and potatoes, and simmer for another 10 minutes. Then add the zucchini and chickpeas, and cook for another 10 minutes.

Pour 2 cups (475 ml) of water into a medium saucepan and bring to a boil over high heat. Remove from heat. Add the couscous, the remaining ½ teaspoon salt, stir, and cover. Allow to stand for 5 minutes, or until all water is absorbed. Add butter and fluff the couscous with a fork.

When the lamb and vegetables are done cooking, taste and adjust seasoning, if necessary.

Serve over hot couscous.

Gluten-Free Alternative:
Substitute 4 cups (696 g) of cooked millet for the couscous in this recipe. Serve the lamb and vegetables on top.

Mediterranean Tradition
Lamb has only 175 calories per 3-ounce (85 g) serving, making it a lean, yet nutrient-rich meat choice. While people in the Mediterranean region don't eat lamb daily, it is a delicious and healthful weekly indulgence that makes a great alternative to fattier beef.

Arabian Rice and Lamb Skillet/
Ouzi "sahla wa sooreya"

Ouzi is prepared in hundreds of different ways across the Arabian Peninsula. It usually consists of whole lambs that are stuffed by the community and roasted over open spits, and enjoyed at holidays. Lamb, rice, and various spices are the common denominators in all of the recipes. I invented this quick and easy weekday version, which can be eaten alone or with a salad on any occasion.

3 tablespoons (45 ml) olive oil, divided

¼ cup (35 g) pine nuts

½ cup (62 g) pistachios, skinned and chopped

1 small onion, diced

1 pound (455 g) lamb fillet, cut into ½-inch (1.3 cm) cubes

1½ cups (315 g) white basmati rice, rinsed, soaked in water for 20 minutes, and drained

2½ cups (570 ml) Vegetable or Chicken Stock (see page 183)

1 teaspoon ground cinnamon

Unrefined sea salt or salt, to taste

Freshly ground pepper, to taste

¼ cup (35 g) raisins

Yield: 4 to 6 servings

Heat 2 tablespoons (30 ml) of oil in a large saucepan over medium heat. Add the nuts, stir, and fry until they begin to color and release their aroma, 30 to 60 seconds. Using a slotted spoon, remove the nuts from the oil.

Add the remaining tablespoon (15 ml) of oil. Add the onion to the pan and sauté until it is translucent, 3 to 5 minutes. Add the lamb meat and brown on all sides. Add rice, stock, cinnamon, salt, and pepper, and stir to incorporate well. Increase heat to high and bring to a boil. Stir and reduce heat to the lowest setting possible. Allow to cook for 20 to 30 minutes, until all liquid is absorbed.

Remove the lid, take off heat, and carefully stir in the nuts, and raisins. Place the lid back on the pan to keep the ouzi warm until serving. If not serving immediately, wrap towels around the saucepan to prevent heat from escaping. If the rice cools before it is time to serve, heat the saucepan over a larger pan filled with hot water to touch the bottom of the rice pan until the rice becomes warm again, or place the rice pan directly over a low flame to reheat.

Mediterranean Tradition
Although this recipe calls for fresh meat, leftover lamb, chicken, beef, or veal pieces can also be transformed into an elegant dinner when added to this recipe. Fried nuts make a rich, nutritious, and crunchy garnish for rice dishes, salads, and soups.

Turkish Eggplant and Herbed Rice Pilaf/
Patlicanli Pilav

Pilafs are believed to have originated in Central Asia millennia ago. It is said that the word *plov* or pilaf, comes from the ancient Greek word *poluv*, or "varied mixture." The name dates back to the days of Alexander the Great's campaign in the Caucasus. He instructed a soldier to cook a tasty dish from local ingredients that traveled well, and shortly thereafter he was presented with a glorious pilaf. This satisfying and highly fragrant recipe contains most of my favorite ingredients—olive oil, eggplant, nuts, tomatoes, raisins, with savory herbs and sweet spices. I love serving it with braised chicken or meat.

1 pound (455 g) eggplant, cut into 1-inch (2.5 cm) cubes

1/3 cup (80 ml) good-quality olive oil, divided

1 large onion, finely chopped

3 tablespoons (27 g) pine nuts or blanched almonds

2 medium ripe tomatoes, peeled and chopped

1 teaspoon unrefined sea salt or salt

Freshly ground black pepper

1 teaspoon pure cinnamon

½ teaspoon allspice

2 tablespoons (8 g) chopped fresh parsley

2 tablespoons (8 g) chopped fresh dill

1½ cups (355 ml) Vegetable or Chicken Stock (see page 183) or water

1 cup (185 g) white basmati rice, soaked in cold water to cover for 20 minutes and drained

Yield: 4 servings

Preheat the broiler. Place the eggplant on a baking sheet lined with aluminum foil. Pour ¼ cup (60 ml) of olive oil over the top and mix well to coat. Place the eggplant under the broiler and broil until light golden and soft, about 3 minutes, paying close attention so they don't burn. Remove from the oven and set aside.

Add the remaining olive oil to a large saucepan with a fitting lid. Add the onion and sauté 3 to 5 minutes, or until translucent. Stir in the nuts and sauté just until they change color.

Add the tomatoes, salt, pepper, cinnamon, allspice, parsley, dill, and reserved eggplant. Stir in stock or water and increase heat to high. Bring to a boil. Add the rice to the mixture and stir. Reduce heat to low. Place two paper towels over the top of the saucepan. Cover, and simmer for 20 to 30 minutes, or until rice is tender and stock has been absorbed.

Taste, adjust seasonings if necessary, and transfer to a heated serving platter.

Mediterranean Tradition
A Turkish chef once told me that no professional cook would be taken seriously if he didn't know at least forty different ways to cook eggplant. The vegetable is high in fiber, vitamins, and minerals while low in carbohydrates—making it a great choice for those watching their weight. Once a cheap meat substitute for the poor, eggplant is now making a comeback in upscale restaurants. Try roasting or grilling fresh eggplant in advance to add to salads, sandwiches, and pasta recipes.

Spanish Seafood Paella/*Arroz en paella*

Paella is known as *Arroz en Paella* in its homeland of Spain. Original paella recipes consisted of rabbit, chicken, snails, and beans, the paella pans were rubbed in ash and cooked over orange wood. This "party in a pot" is said to be a descendant of Arabian *kabsah,* a similar dish originating in the Arabian Peninsula. Arabs introduced rice into southern Spain in the ninth century, along with spices such as saffron. A unique feature of paella is that a crunchy topping forms on it. Do not worry, this is called the *socarrat* in Valencian dialect, and is the most treasured part of the paella.

2 tablespoons (30 ml) extra-virgin olive oil

1 yellow onion, diced

2 tablespoons (32 g) tomato paste

¼ pound (115 g) jumbo shrimp, deveined and peeled

1 pound (455 g) baby squid, cleaned, peeled, and sliced into rings

¼ pound (115 g) boneless white fish fillet (such as cod or swai), cut into 2-inch (5 cm) pieces

2 cups (390 g) medium-grain Spanish rice

Pinch of good-quality saffron

2 teaspoons sweet paprika

1 clove garlic, minced

2 tablespoons (8 g) Italian parsley

5 cups (1 L) Seafood Stock (see page 183)

1 teaspoon kosher salt

¼ cup (45 g) jarred pimiento peppers

Yield: 8 servings

Heat the oil in a large wide skillet over medium heat. Add the onion and cook until golden brown, about 5 minutes. Add the tomato paste, and stir slowly to heat through and blend the paste with onion and oil.

Add the shrimp, squid, and fish to the pan. Cook until barely opaque, 3 to 5 minutes. Add the rice and stir in the saffron, paprika, garlic, and parsley. Pour the stock over the top of the mixture and add salt.

Increase heat to high and bring to a boil, reduce heat to low, and stir. Cook the paella, uncovered for 30 to 40 minutes, or until all liquid is absorbed, stirring occasionally.

When the paella is done, allow to stand at room temperature for 10 minutes. Garnish with pimientos and serve warm.

Mediterranean Tradition
Saffron and paprika are used heavily in Spain. The benefits of paprika include increasing saliva production, easing digestion, regulating blood pressure, and improving circulation by providing a blood thinning agent. It also contains high levels of vitamin C. Saffron contains a high amount of antioxidants known to prevent disease. Try using paprika and saffron to flavor potatoes, rice, pasta, soups, and stews.

Cannellini Bean, Barley, and Tomato Soup/
Zuppa di cannellini, orzo e pomodori

My favorite way of making tomato soup is to start with a traditional Italian tomato sauce as a base. When making that recipe, you can make a double batch of the sauce and reserve half of it before using the remainder to make this soup. In a pinch, you can use a good-quality, low-sodium jarred tomato sauce to make the recipe. Note that dried beans need to be soaked overnight. A 15.5-ounce (440 g) can of reduced-sodium beans that have been drained and rinsed could be substituted.

1 tablespoon (15 ml) extra-virgin olive oil

3 cloves garlic, minced

1 cup (250 g) tomato purée

Kosher salt

Freshly ground pepper

¼ cup (15 g) freshly chopped parsley or basil

1 cup (177 g) dried cannellini beans, covered in hot water overnight, and drained

3 cups (710 ml) Vegetable or Chicken Stock (see page 183)

½ cup (100 g) pearl barley

¼ cup (30 g) grated Pecorino Romano cheese

Yield: 4 servings

Heat oil in a large saucepan over medium heat.

Add garlic and sauté until it releases its aroma, about 1 minute. Add tomato purée, salt, and pepper.

Increase heat to high and bring to a boil. Add parsley or basil and cannellini beans. Stir, reduce heat to low, and cover. Simmer for 15 minutes.

Remove the lid carefully, and stir in the stock. Bring to a boil, uncovered, over high heat. Reduce heat to low, stir in the barley, and cook 10 to 15 minutes until the barley is al dente.

Garnish with cheese and serve hot.

> **Mediterranean Tradition**
> Cannelini, or white kidney, beans have a very low glycemic index, making them an excellent choice for those with diabetes, and anyone trying to lose weight and gain muscle. They have also been proven to prevent colorectal cancer and have an overall detoxifying effect on the body. These beans make a great addition to soups, stews and salads. Pearl barley has had the hull and bran layers removed before it is polished, giving it the pearl name.

Quinoa, Arugula, and Fig Salad/
Salade de Quinoa, Roquette e Figues

This French spin on tabbouleh replaces bulgur wheat with nutritious quinoa—the ancient grain that supplies all nine essential amino acids, making it a complete protein! If fresh figs are not in season, substitute pears, apples, oranges, or the fruit of your choice. In addition to being used in this salad, cooked quinoa tastes great at breakfast with fruit, cinnamon, chopped nuts, and milk.

1 cup (185 g) dry quinoa, rinsed

½ cup (118 ml) extra-virgin olive oil

Juice of 1 lemon

¼ teaspoon unrefined sea salt or salt

Black pepper, to taste

1 pint (228 g) fresh figs, quartered

11 ounces (312 g) baby arugula

Yield: 4 servings as a vegetarian main, or 8 as a side dish

Bring 2 cups (475 ml) of water to a boil in a medium saucepan over high heat. Add the quinoa, stir, reduce heat to low, and cover. Allow to simmer until all liquid is absorbed, 10 to 15 minutes. Remove from the stove and allow to cool completely. Whisk the olive oil, lemon juice, salt, and black pepper together to form vinaigrette.

Place the quinoa in a large bowl and lightly fluff with a fork. Combine with the vinaigrette. Gently stir in figs. Place the arugula on a platter. Pour the quinoa mixture over the arugula and serve.

Mediterranean Tradition
A new trend in the Mediterranean region is to use quinoa instead of rice in traditional recipes. Try adding cooked quinoa to soups, beans, and stews to increase their nutritional value. You can also use cooked quinoa as a bed for main courses. A terrific variation on this salad substitutes the juice of 1 orange for the lemon, and 2 cups (454 g) fresh berries and 11 ounces (312 g) baby spinach for the figs and arugula.

Whole-Wheat Fusilli with Almond-Arugula Pesto/
Fusilli integrali con pesto di mandorle e rucola

This easy-to-prepare pasta is packed with as much flavor as it is nutrients. While traditional pasta is best prepared in summer when fresh basil is at its finest, this version can be enjoyed all year long. The pesto also tastes great slathered over roasted salmon or tossed with cooked baby potatoes.

1 pound (455 g) whole-wheat fusilli or any short quinoa pasta

3 cups (60 g) fresh baby arugula

2 cloves garlic

¼ cup (36 g) blanched almonds

¼ cup (60 ml) good-quality extra-virgin olive oil (unfiltered, if possible)

¼ cup (25 g) grated Parmigiano-Reggiano cheese

¼ cup (30 g) grated Pecorino Romano cheese

1 pint (230 g) cherry tomatoes, halved

Yield: 6 to 8 servings

Cook the pasta according to package directions, until al dente. Drain, reserving ½ cup (120 ml) of pasta water.

Combine the arugula, garlic, and almonds in a food processor. Process until chopped while pouring olive oil into the processor. Add some pasta water if necessary to thin out.

Spoon the pesto into a medium bowl. Stir in the Parmigiano and Pecorino cheeses. Stir the pesto into the pasta and add in cherry tomatoes. Mix well to combine and serve.

Mediterranean Tradition
I mention arugula many times in this book—and for good reason! A peasant staple since antiquity in the Mediterranean region, it is packed with folic acid, Vitamins A, C, and K, iron, and copper, making it a powerful protector against cancer and an excellent choice for enhancing brain function. It also has cooling and hydrating effects on the body, making it a great choice for those in warmer climates. Try swapping regular lettuce for arugula in your favorite recipes.

Whole-Wheat Orecchiete Pasta with Broccoli and Garlic/
Orecchiete integrale con broccoli

Orecchiete, or "little ears," are popular, artisanal pasta shapes in the southern Italian regions of Basilicata, Puglia, and Calabria. This dish is one of the most classic ways to prepare them. I've replaced the dried white pasta available in the United States with whole wheat in this recipe, for enhanced nutritional benefits. It is important to note, however, that in its native regions in Italy, the wheat used to make pasta is *grano duro,* which is more nutritious.

⅓ cup (80 ml) good-quality, cold-pressed olive oil, preferably Puglian

3 cloves garlic, finely chopped

½ chile pepper, minced, or ½ teaspoon crushed red chili flakes

¼ cup (35 g) pine nuts

12 small cherry tomatoes, quartered

½ teaspoon unrefined sea salt or salt

¼ teaspoon fresh-ground black pepper

½ pound (225 g) broccoli florets

2 tablespoons (5 g) freshly chopped basil or Italian parsley

1 pound (455 g) whole-wheat orecchiette, or any short rice pasta

¼ cup (30 g) grated Pecorino Romano cheese, for serving

Yield: 6 servings

Heat the olive oil in a large, wide skillet over medium heat. Add the garlic and chile pepper and sauté about 1 minute, just until they release their aroma. Add the pine nuts and sauté until lightly golden. Add the cherry tomatoes, salt, and pepper. Stir, and cook for 2 minutes.

Add the broccoli florets, basil or parsley, and ½ cup (120 ml) water, stir, and cover. Cook until the broccoli is fork-tender, 10 to 15 minutes.

Meanwhile cook the pasta in a large pot of slightly salted boiling water for about 12 minutes, or until al dente. Drain, and add to the finished sauce. Toss to combine. Taste and adjust seasonings, if necessary. Top with Pecorino Romano cheese.

Mediterranean Tradition
Save the unused broccoli stems from this recipe to use as additions to soup, or try boiling and puréeing them. Then mix with a little bit of Pecorino cheese and olive oil for a delicious and nutritious side dish.

Whole-Wheat Country Moroccan Bread/*Khubz Baladi*

This easy bread, often made with barley, has a soft, moist crumb. It is a Moroccan recipe, and it's a great bread for any meal. It is best eaten the day it is made, or frozen then defrosted and reheated the day it is served. Freeze by wrapping it in plastic wrap and then aluminum foil. Thaw at room temperature and warm in a preheated 350°F (180°C) oven before serving.

2½ cups (570 ml) warm water

1 tablespoon (12 g) active, dry yeast

2 teaspoons sugar

1 teaspoon kosher salt

6 to 8 cups (750 g to 1kg) whole-wheat or barley flour, plus extra for kneading (see Gluten-Free Alternative)

4 teaspoons (20 ml) extra-virgin olive oil, divided

3 teaspoons (8 g) sesame seeds

Yield: 3 round loaves

Pour the warm water into the bowl of a standing electric mixer with a paddle attachment. Sprinkle the yeast and sugar over the water, and mix until dissolved. Add the salt and gradually mix in 6 cups (750 g) of flour, adding up to 2 more cups, one cup (125 g) at a time, until dough pulls away from the side of the bowl. Switch to a hook attachment and knead for 5 minutes on medium speed, or until smooth. Roll the dough into a 12-inch (30 cm) log, then divide into three equal pieces. Shape each piece into a 4-inch (10 cm) dome-shaped loaf. Place loaves on a baking sheet greased with 1 teaspoon oil. Cover with a kitchen towel and place in a draft-free area to rise for 1 hour, or until doubled.

Preheat the oven to 350°F (180°C). Uncover the loaves and brush each with 1 teaspoon olive oil and 1 teaspoon sesame seeds. Bake for 20 to 30 minutes, or until lightly golden. Let cool slightly, and serve warm.

Gluten-Free Alternative:
Replace whole-wheat flour with a combination of 3 to 5 cups (474 to 790 g) brown rice flour, 1 cup (125 g) tapioca flour, 2 cups (272 g) sorghum flour, and 2 teaspoons xanthan gum.

Mediterranean Tradition
One of the earliest cultivated grains, barley is a member of the grass family and has been cultivated since the ninth millennia BCE. Its production boomed after the second millennia BCE in Mesopotamia, and it became a popular, inexpensive, and nutritious ingredient in the Mediterranean region. Containing eight essential amino acids, barley has been widely used in many cultures and has been proven to regulate blood sugar levels.

FRUITS

When I think of my time spent in various places in the Mediterranean, fruit is one of the first things that comes to mind. It is such an integral part of the culture that it's difficult not to get swept away by its sensual appeal. Fresh, local, seasonal, and often organic, the fruits of the region are culinary jewels begging to be savored. I have my favorites in each country, and, believe it or not, often make travel plans depending on the fruit harvests!

I can't imagine my life in Italy without thinking of fresh figs. My landlady in Rome used to bring me plates of them from her tree—a definite perk to living in her building! The southern Italian region of Calabria, my ancestral homeland, is famous for its figs. After the harvest, thousands of fresh figs are decked out on wooden planks to dry in the sun. Later, they are transformed into sweet and savory cookies, preserves, bread, cakes, and more.

In Egypt, where I've spent a great deal of time, as well as in the rest of North Africa, early spring is orange season. Take a drive near an orange orchard, and you can smell the thick, musky citrus scent from about a mile (1.6 km) before you can even see the trees. The smell is so intoxicating that when I return home, I often find myself sniffing and sipping orange blossom water, just to be transported back to that magical place.

In the North African and Middle Eastern regions of the Mediterranean, October is date season. Fresh dates taste nothing like the dried supermarket varieties that we get in the United States, no matter how great the quality is. There are scores of fresh date varieties to choose from, and they usually are ruby or amber colored, about the size of a large jalapeño pepper, and have a slightly fibrous texture like celery. Their flavor is similar to an apple, yet more complex. Many countries have date festivals where the whole community gathers to harvest the dates, and they are transformed into date breads, cookies, molasses, puddings, and more.

My affection for fruit is not unique. Everyone who hails from the region feels the same way. Since antiquity, communities relied on fresh fruit not only as a culinary ingredient, but often as a trading commodity. Entire villages and towns would (and often still do) celebrate the harvests of grapes, oranges, figs, dates, cherries, apples, pears, peaches, pomegranates, persimmons, and other fruits. In addition to their entertainment value, these festivals also played an important role in the marketing of fruit and fruit products. By demonstrating dozens of ways in which fruits and other culinary ingredients could be used, high levels of fruit consumption became second nature.

Most of these fruits are native to the region, while others, such as melons and peaches, were introduced via the Silk Road trading with Central Asia. While the Silk Road commerce is often associated with spices and textiles alone, many foods and cooking methods were exchanged as well. The great civilizations of China, India, Egypt, Persia, Rome, and Arabia were fortified by the powerful commercial ties that the route provided from approximately 500 BCE to 1500 CE.

Nutritional Benefits

The high amount of fiber and other nutrients in fruit make it the perfect food for people on the go. According to Catherine Itsiopoulos, A.P.D., A.N., head of the Department of Dietetics and Human Nutrition at La Trobe University in Melbourne, who has conducted numerous research studies on the Mediterranean diet, "fresh fruit should be eaten daily," and "dried fruit and nuts should be consumed as snacks and desserts."

Studies conducted around the globe for decades have shown that consuming a diet high in fruits and vegetables lowers risks for chronic illnesses, including cancer and cardiovascular disease. Until recently, however, it was difficult to determine exactly how those already suffering from heart disease could improve their health with the diet. But a landmark 2013 study conducted by Dr. Ramon Estruch, a professor of medicine at the University of Barcelona, proves that heart disease can be reduced by 30 percent by following a Mediterranean diet consisting of balanced meals with fruits, vegetables, and olive oil.

The National Center for Chronic Disease Prevention and Health Promotion has also proven that a diet high in fruits and vegetables may help people to manage their weight, in addition to lowering risk for chronic diseases and improving overall health. According to researchers, the water and fiber in fruits increase volume and therefore reduce energy density of the food. This is important because foods with high energy density have a high number of calories per weight of food, and cause weight gain. Fruits make you feel fuller faster with fewer calories. The study also illustrated the importance of dietary fiber in weight regulation. Whole fruit not only contains more fiber because of the peel, but it is considered lower in energy density (calories per weight) and more fulfilling than fruit juices, making it the top choice, when available.

The recipes that follow are for fruit-based snacks, breakfasts, and desserts. Let your imagination be your guide and challenge yourself to incorporate mouthwatering fruit into each of your meals.

Seasonal Fruit Platter

Ripe fresh fruit, enjoyed at its peak, can be so hard to come by that it is preferred over elaborate, decadent desserts. This recipe calls for a selection of summer fruits, but that doesn't mean that a fruit platter can't be served all year long. In most countries in the Mediterranean, fresh fruit completes a meal. Whether it's a plate of fresh oranges in the spring, fresh figs, dates, and grapes in the fall, or apples and pears in the winter, their flavor can't be beat. Eating seasonal fruits is healthier because they contain the nutrients our bodies need during that specific time of year.

2 cups (290 g) fresh strawberries

1 cup (145 g) chopped fresh cantaloupe

1 cup (180 g) chopped fresh honeydew melon

1 cup (165 g) chopped fresh pineapple (peeled, cored and diced into 1-inch, or 2.5 cm, wedges)

8 kiwi, peeled and sliced into ¼-inch rounds (6 mm)

Yield: 6 servings

Arrange the fruit in a pleasing pattern on a serving plate and serve with cocktail forks or cocktail toothpicks.

Mediterranean Tradition

Local, fresh fruit is easier to come by in many Mediterranean countries than it is elsewhere. For a long-term health investment, plant your own fruit trees or gardens. Even if you don't have a lot of space, some fruits, like strawberries, can be grown in containers on a terrace or balcony. By growing your own fruit, you'll save time and money while eating healthier.

Spanish Dried Fruit, Nut, and Cheese Platter/
Plato de frutas secas, nueces y queso

Dried fruits are nutrient-dense and a particularly good source of dietary fiber, potassium, and phenolic compounds, which are linked to a number of health benefits, including decreased risk of heart disease, diabetes, and certain types of cancer. In a study by the Harvard School of Public Health, researchers found a significant decrease in weight associated with an increased consumption of nuts. Furthermore, eating just a handful of nuts a day may help curb your appetite.

1 wedge (about 8 ounces, or 225 g) Manchego cheese

1 wedge (about 8 ounces, or 225 g) Cabrales cheese

1 wedge (about 6 ounces, or 170 g) goat cheese

1 bunch seedless red grapes

1 bunch seedless green grapes

1 cup (178 g) dried Medjool dates

1 cup (130 g) dried apricots

8 dried figs

1 cup (145 g) blanched almonds, toasted

Yield: 8 servings

Arrange the cheeses together on a very large platter.

Arrange the fresh and dried fruits, and almonds around the cheese on the platter. Or, arrange the fruit and nuts on another platter.

Mediterranean Tradition
Las doce uvas de la suerte, or "the twelve grapes of luck," is a Spanish tradition dating back to the nineteenth century that involves eating a grape with each stroke of the clock at midnight on New Year's Eve to ensure a prosperous new year. In addition to their folkloric appeal, grapes offer a great deal of nutritional benefits including vitamins A, C, B$_6$, folate, selenium, magnesium, potassium, calcium, iron, and phosphorus. Flavanoids found in grapes are strong antioxidants which are believed to slow down aging. Grown in the Mediterranean region since antiquity, grapes are a fantastic addition to daily meal plans.

North African Fruit "Cocktail"/*Assir Fawakha Taza*

Countries from Morocco to Egypt and Turkey serve fresh fruit cocktails at street-side fruit stands. Decorated with hanging bags of ripe, fresh, seasonal fruit, they offer some of the most delicious, but fortunately not guilty, pleasures to be had. Feel free to substitute your favorite fruit trio whenever the mood strikes.

1 pound (455 g) strawberries, cleaned and trimmed

¼ cup (50 g) sugar, or to taste

1 cup (235 ml) fresh orange juice

4 teaspoons (20 ml) pomegranate or other syrup

16 pomegranate arils (seeds)

Yield: 4 cocktails

Chill 4 clear glasses. Purée the strawberries in a blender until frothy. Add sugar, to taste, and whip until combined. Divide the strawberry juice equally among the 4 glasses.

Holding the back of a spoon over the strawberry juice, pour the orange juice over the top of the spoon (this prevents the two colors from mixing). Repeat with the other three glasses.

Pour 1 teaspoon of pomegranate syrup on top of each glass and garnish each with a few pomegranate seeds. Serve immediately.

Mediterranean Tradition
Even though these sweet fruit drinks are made in a few minutes, they are not considered a fast food. Most people stop to enjoy a fruit cocktail as part of an evening stroll with family and friends, reinforcing the popular Mediterranean trends of walking and enjoying fresh fruit after a meal, which is a healthful alternative to ice cream and TV. Look for pomegranate syrup, a condensed pomegranate juice, in Mediterranean markets.

Strawberry "Beauty" Smoothie

If you're looking for a beauty boost, this sweet and satisfying smoothie is just for you! Strawberries are a great way to get more fiber, vitamin C, and healthy cancer-preventing compounds into your diet. Bananas are rich in vitamin A, B, and E, making them powerful antiaging agents that are often applied directly on the skin as masks. The presence of live cultures along with lactic acid, zinc, and other minerals and enzymes in yogurt make it a great choice for improving skin condition as well. Flaxseed was cultivated in Babylon as early as 3000 BCE and contains a high amount of omega-3 fatty acids, which can help lower cholesterol and improve the complexion.

1 very ripe banana, sliced

1 cup (100 g) ice

1 cup (230 g) yogurt

2 tablespoons (40 g) organic honey, or to taste

1 cup (145 g) strawberries

2 tablespoons (24 g) flaxseeds

Yield: 2 servings

Blend the banana, ice, yogurt, and honey together until the banana is well blended. Add the strawberries and flaxseeds and blend on low speed for 30 seconds or until frothy. Pour into clear glasses and serve cold.

Mediterranean Tradition
Traditionally, many facial and skin care regimens in the Mediterranean region utilized fruits as their primary ingredients. Try combining yogurt with honey and applying it over dry skin. Leave on for 20 minutes, rinse, and dry. Your skin will be extremely soft and supple.

Apricot and Orange Blossom Pudding with Pistachios/
Mahallabiya Qamr Din bil Mahazar wa Fusdooq

Dairy-free fruit puddings such as this one make sweet, light, and satisfying finales to any meal. Orange blossom water can be found in Mediterranean and Middle Eastern markets, or in the baking aisle of gourmet grocery stores.

1 pound (455 g) dried apricots

1 cup (200 g) sugar

4 tablespoons (32 g) cornstarch dissolved in ¼ cup (60 ml) cold water

1 tablespoon (15 ml) orange blossom water

Handful of pistachios, shelled and finely chopped

Yield: 8 servings

Chop the apricots into small pieces. Place them in a large bowl and cover them with 4 cups (950 ml) of boiling water. Cover the bowl with a plate or lid. When the apricot pieces break down and nearly dissolve, add the sugar, and stir. Purée the mixture in a blender.

Pour the apricot juice into a medium saucepan. Add the cornstarch mixture and stir well with a wooden spoon to combine. Set the heat to high and allow the mixture to boil for 2 minutes, stirring constantly. Reduce heat to medium-low, add the orange blossom water, and continue cooking the pudding, stirring slowly until it thickens and pulls away from the sides of the saucepan.

Pour into individual ramekins or a large decorative bowl. Sprinkle pistachios on top in a pattern and refrigerate about 2 hours, or until set. Serve cold.

Mediterranean Tradition
If you ever drive through the Mediterranean countryside in March or April, a thick musky, citrus aroma might start to overwhelm your senses. After a mile or two (1.6 or 3.2 km), you will pass an orange orchard. In many areas of the Mediterranean, that very scent gets preserved for year-round use in a lovely ingredient called orange blossom water. The distilled essential oils from the orange blossoms themselves get transformed into a heady, intoxicating liquid that enhances everything with just a single drop. Used in everything from Middle Eastern baklavas to French clafoutis and Neapolitan *Pastiera* cakes, some people even iron their linens with it.

Poached Vanilla-Scented Pears and Figs/
Pere alla vaniglia con ficchi secchi

This dessert is so elegant and delicious that no one will even realize that it's good for them! Pears are a great source of dietary fiber, which lowers cholesterol and prevents colon cancer. Ounce per ounce, figs, one of the world's oldest fruits, contain more nutrients than any other fruit.

4 Bosc pears, peeled

16 dried figs

2 tablespoons (30 ml) lemon juice

2 tablespoons (40 g) honey

1 teaspoon pure vanilla bean paste or pure vanilla extract

Yield: 4 servings

Slice off the bottoms of the pears so they can stand firmly. Place the pears and figs in a medium saucepan and cover with water.

Add the lemon juice, honey, and vanilla paste. Bring to a boil over high heat, reduce heat to medium-low, and simmer 20 minutes, or until the pears are tender.

When the pears are cool enough to handle, remove them from the poaching liquid and stand them upright in the middle of 4 dessert plates.

Drizzle a few tablespoons of cooking liquid over the tops of the pears and arrange 4 figs around the sides of each plate.

Allow to stand for 5 minutes at room temperature and serve.

Mediterranean Tradition
Getting family and friends involved in preparing meals is a Mediterranean tradition worth copying. In addition to making the work easier and more pleasurable, the communal aspect of sharing a task is emotionally satisfying. In addition, you'll be less likely to order unhealthy take-out if you know that others are looking forward to cooking.

Rose- and Mint-Infused Fruit Salad/
Salata Fawakha bil Meya Ward wa Na'na

I love the way rose water perks up the flavor of berries and melon. I first tasted this recipe at a royal palace in Saudi Arabia. It was served as part of a truly ornate afternoon tea service. Use whatever fresh fruit is available to make this delicious fruit salad. The fruit may be chopped the day before serving, stored in the refrigerator, and then tossed to combine at least five hours, or the night before serving, to allow the rose and mint flavors to blend properly.

1 cup (170 g) cubed cantaloupe

½ cup (65 g) raspberries

½ cup (75 g) strawberries

½ cup (75 g) blueberries

½ cup (89 g) sliced kiwi

¼ cup (50 g) sugar

1 teaspoon rose water

4 tablespoons (24 g) finely chopped fresh mint

4 teaspoons (20 g) yogurt, for garnish (optional)

Yield: 4 servings

Combine all of the fruit in a large salad bowl. Mix the sugar, rose water, and mint together in a small bowl.

Drizzle the sugar mixture over fruit and mix gently to combine.

Cover the bowl, and store in refrigerator for a minimum of 5 hours or maximum overnight.

Transfer to individual bowls before serving. Garnish with yogurt, if desired.

> **Mediterranean Tradition**
> Rose water is one of the most unique and delicious ingredients in the Mediterranean. It can perk up the flavor of everything from fruit to drinks. It is made from the distillation of rose oil. After Islamic alchemists perfected distillation, rose water became an indispensable ingredient in drinks and desserts everywhere from Turkey in the eastern Mediterranean to Morocco in the West. It is also a popular cosmetic ingredient, used as a facial toner or mixed with dried ground lemon peels in facial masks. Look for rose water in organic and Mediterranean markets.

Grilled Peaches with Frozen Yogurt and Honey/
Pesche alla griglia con gelato di yogurt e miele

Peaches originated in Central Asia and made their way to the Mediterranean via Silk Route trading. Any type of peach can be used to make this recipe provided that they are ripe, but not too soft. The grill's sizzling heat instantly sears the surface of the fruit upon contact, which caramelizes its sugars and enhances its natural sweetness. Frozen Greek yogurt, full of inulin, which helps balance blood sugar levels, and healing honey, complement the peach flavors perfectly.

4 medium ripe peaches, cut in half (pits removed)

1 cup (245 g) plain frozen Greek yogurt

8 tablespoons (160 g) honey

Cinnamon

Yield: 4 servings

Place the peaches cut-side down on the grill. Grill on low or indirect heat until soft, 2 to 4 minutes on each side.

Set the peaches on a serving platter and top each with 2 tablespoons (31 g) of frozen Greek yogurt.

Drizzle a tablespoon (20 g) of honey over the top of each and garnish with a dash of cinnamon. Serve immediately.

> **Mediterranean Tradition**
> Always make more grilled fruit than you need for your recipe. It tastes great cut up and tossed into salads and pilafs, and it is a quick, easy way to pack extra nutrients into a meal.

Italian Baked Apples with Cream and Amaretti/
Mele al forno con crema ed amaretti

There are more than 7,000 varieties of apples in the United States alone, yet most of those available to consumers fall within one of 50 varieties. The apple was cultivated in ancient Egypt. There are many mythological associations over various civilizations, with the apple in the Garden of Eden being the most widely known. Throughout the Middle Ages in the eastern Mediterranean, people gave an apple with a bite out of it to their romantic interests. This classic Italian recipe is easy enough to be enjoyed anytime, but elegant enough for entertaining.

1 tablespoon (14 g) butter

6 apples, cored

1 cup (236 ml) heavy cream, divided

¼ cup (50 g) sugar

6 ounces (170 ml) amaretti, or other gluten-free cookies

Yield: 6 servings

Preheat the oven to 350°F (180°C) and grease a 9-inch (23 cm) baking pan with butter.

Place the apples in the baking pan and add water to a depth of ⅛ inch (3 mm). Place in the oven and bake, uncovered, until the apples are tender but still firm, about half an hour. Remove from the oven and let cool.

Heat ½ cup (118 ml) of cream and the sugar in a medium saucepan over medium heat until boiling, stirring with a wooden spoon. When the sugar has dissolved, set aside to cool for 5 minutes.

Whip the remaining ½ cup (118 ml) cream until firm. Reserve half of the whipped cream for decorating. With a spatula, fold the remaining ¼ cup whipped cream into the cooled cream and sugar mixture.

Arrange the apples in a deep serving dish. Pour cream sauce over them and pipe the reserved whipped cream around them. Crumble the amaretti cookies and sprinkle over the tops of apples.

Mediterranean Tradition

The high fiber content in apples makes them a rich source of soluble fiber, which helps prevent a build-up of cholesterol in blood vessels and reduces the risk of heart attack. Apple peels are especially good choices for diabetics because they help to slow down the rate that sugar is absorbed in the blood. In addition to being eaten raw, apples are a great alternative to potatoes in stews, taste great in salads, and make fantastic desserts.

Roasted Plums with Basil-Yogurt Cream/
Susine al forno con yogurt e basilico

Roasting fruits enhances their sweetness and gives them a unique texture. Serving them with yogurt and herbs increases health benefits. Keep this in mind when planning desserts for yourself, friends, and family. Even though recipes such as these are simple and healthful, many people prefer their flavor to store-bought cakes and pastries.

1 teaspoon olive oil

4 ripe plums, halved and pitted

4 teaspoons (16 g) sugar

1 cup (230 g) vanilla yogurt

2 tablespoons (5 g) finely chopped fresh basil

1 teaspoon honey

Yield: 4 servings

Preheat the oven to 400°F (200°C). Oil a large baking dish. Place the plums inside, cut side up, and sprinkle ½ teaspoon sugar over each. Bake, uncovered, for 35 minutes.

While the plums are baking, stir together the yogurt, basil, and honey.

Divide half of yogurt mixture onto each of 4 plates, or a large serving platter.

When plums are finished baking, remove them from the oven and place 2 halves over yogurt on each plate. Fill the holes with remaining yogurt mixture and serve warm.

Mediterranean Tradition
If you're prone to skipping breakfast, prepare larger quantities of dishes such as this one in the evening. The fiber-rich plums and the protein-packed yogurt will keep you pleasantly full for hours.

VEGETABLES

When organic vegetables are ripe and in season, or cooked to perfection—with their natural sugars coaxed out of them and combined with other savory ingredients—eating healthfully becomes a labor of love. It's one of the reasons why the Mediterranean diet is so popular.

Agrarian festivals were celebrated in many parts of the region since antiquity. In Italy, those festivals are called *sagre*, or "sacred," and they are still held today. Originally held in honor of the gods, they now commemorate the harvest of a particular food and may be combined with a patron saint; other times they are celebrated specifically for their culinary attributes. In ancient Rome, there were 182 sacred days, many of them with their own foods.

Today there are hundreds of *sagre* for garlic, wild asparagus, fennel, prickly pears, chile peppers, white truffles, cheese, tomatoes, onions, and more. During the festivals, farmers, chefs, housewives, artisan producers, and entertainers provide their services for members of the community. Whole families gather for what have become some of the most important social events on the calendar. Children growing up in an environment such as this are fortunate because, just by attending a *sagre,* they are exposed to vegetables prepared in countless ways—and they receive a valuable culinary education at a very young age.

Italy, however, is not alone in its ingenious use of vegetables. The art of being able to prepare a single vegetable in numerous ways is prized throughout the region. In Turkey, for example, there is a legend surrounding the dish *Imam Biyaldi,* or "The Imam Fainted." Legend has it that once upon a time an honorable Imam who was also an eligible bachelor wanted to choose a wife. The single women of the town lined up to meet him. Each woman who stood before the Imam, known to be a fan of eggplant, was asked to prepare as many eggplant dishes as she could. One of the women prepared forty, including the Imam Biyaldi—which was apparently so intoxicating that it made the Imam faint. Whether the story is true is up for discussion, but it does drive home the point that versatility with vegetables makes a better spouse.

Mediterranean cooks are masters at vegetables, and for good reason. Meals are not planned around protein, as in the United States and western Europe. Cooks in the Mediterranean begin planning a meal based on the produce that is in season. Meat, fish, seafood, poultry, and dairy are thought of as accompaniments, and produce is the foundation of an entire meal.

Home cooks and professional chefs in all regions of the world can take inspiration from their Mediterranean counterparts by first considering which vegetables to prepare. This shift in mindset alone will encourage vegetable intake. In addition to experiencing their great tastes and textures, eating a wide variety of vegetables ensures maximum vitamin and mineral intake, as well as more fiber and less fat in the diet.

Nutritional Benefits

The average American eats only 57 percent of the recommended amount of vegetables daily, and only 6 percent eat the amount that they should. This is a shame because eating vegetables is one of the easiest ways to stay healthy and in shape. We should be consuming four to five different types of fresh vegetables daily, preferably of different colors, to ensure the widest range of nutrients.

Vegetables naturally have high levels of water, making them virtually fat free and low in calories. Consuming vegetables helps to maintain blood pressure levels as well as the digestive, skeletal, and excretory systems. The antioxidants in vegetables help keep cancer, cardiovascular problems and strokes at bay; vegetables deliver vitamins, including folate, vitamin A, vitamin K, and vitamin B_6, as well as antioxidant carotenoids such as beta carotene from carrots, zeaxanthin from greens, and lutein from spinach and collard greens.

Different-colored vegetables provide different nutrients and benefits. Green leafy vegetables, for example, are high in magnesium and a have a low glycemic index, making them especially important for those with type II diabetes. In fact, eating just one serving of green leafy vegetables each day has been shown to lower the risks associated with diabetes.

Vegetables also contain minerals and phenolic flavonoid antioxidants. A deficiency in these particular nutrients can lead to problems with vital organs, bones, and teeth. Quercetin is a bioflavanoid that produces anti-cancer and anti-inflammatory powers of vegetables.

Cabbage, Brussels sprouts, cauliflower, and broccoli have a high content of indoles and isothiocyanates. These components have protective properties against colon cancer, breast cancer, skin cancer, and other types of cancers. Vegetables are also great options for consuming dietary fiber, which makes you feel fuller for longer, preventing overeating and helping to maintain a healthy weight.

Quick Italian Pickles/*Giardiniera*

This traditional Italian method of preserving fresh-from-the-garden vegetables can be made in a flash by following this easy method. Pearl onions and chile peppers can be used as well. They make a great addition to an antipasto platter.

1 cup (235 ml) white wine vinegar

1 cup (235 ml) water

1 tablespoon (13 g) sugar

1 bay leaf

½ + ⅛ teaspoon crushed red pepper, divided, if desired

5 whole black peppercorns

½ + ⅛ teaspoon unrefined sea salt or salt, divided

2 cloves garlic, thinly sliced

1½ cups (150 g) bite-size cauliflower flowerets

1 rib celery, thinly sliced

¾ cup carrot, cut into 1-inch (2.5 cm) rectangular pieces

½ red bell pepper, cut into 1-inch (2.5 cm) pieces

½ green bell pepper, cut into 1-inch (2.5 cm) pieces

1½ tablespoons (23 ml) extra-virgin olive oil

Freshly ground black pepper

Yield: About 2½ cups (380 g)

Combine the vinegar, water, sugar, bay leaf, ½ teaspoon crushed red pepper (if using), black peppercorns, and ½ teaspoon salt in a large saucepan. Bring to a boil.

Add the garlic, cauliflower, celery, carrot, and red and green bell peppers. Reduce heat to maintain a lively simmer and cook until the vegetables are tender-crisp, 3 to 5 minutes. Remove from the heat and let stand for 5 minutes. Reserve 3 tablespoons (45 ml) of the cooking liquid, then drain. Remove the bay leaf.

Transfer the vegetables to a medium bowl. Stir in the oil, pepper, the remaining ⅛ teaspoon each crushed red pepper (if using) and salt and the reserved cooking liquid. Refrigerate for at least 25 minutes to chill. Stir and serve with a slotted spoon.

Mediterranean Tradition
Pickled vegetables are believed to stimulate the appetite, help us to digest food better, and absorb more nutrients from what we are eating. In Naples, Italy, this same vegetable mixture is drained, dressed with olive oil and fresh herbs, and served at the Christmas *cenone* or "big meal."

Greek-Style Stewed Green Beans with Dill/*Fasolia*

This flavorful way of preparing green beans is very popular in Greece. Green beans are a good source of vitamins A and C, and folate. They contain very low acidity, making them a great choice for people on anti-inflammatory diets. This is a quick and tasty way to serve them. They also taste great when added into soups and stews, or blanched and tossed into salads.

1 tablespoon (15 ml) extra-virgin olive oil

1 small yellow onion, diced

4 cloves garlic, chopped

1¾ cups (315 g) diced tomatoes

¼ cup (15 g) finely chopped fresh baby dill

1 teaspoon unrefined sea salt or salt

Freshly ground black pepper

1 pound (455 g) thin, French-style green beans (*haricots verts*), ends trimmed

1 lemon, cut into 8 thin slices

Yield: 8 servings

Heat the olive oil in a medium saucepan over medium heat. Add the onion and sauté until translucent, 3 to 5 minutes. Stir in the garlic and cook for 1 minute.

Stir in the tomatoes, dill, salt, and freshly ground pepper. Bring to a boil over high heat, add the green beans, stir, and reduce heat to low. Simmer for 10 to 15 minutes, or until the green beans are tender. Spoon onto a serving platter and garnish with lemon.

Mediterranean Tradition
Substitute cauliflower, potatoes, or peas in this easy recipe for a quick and unique side dish whenever needed.

Provencal Bistro Carrot Salad/
Salade aux carottes râpées

This is a French bistro classic—simple to prepare, and perfect as a light side dish.

1 teaspoon Dijon mustard

1 tablespoon (15 ml) lemon juice

5 tablespoons (75 ml) extra-virgin olive oil

5 medium carrots, peeled, trimmed, and grated

Unrefined sea salt or salt

Freshly ground black pepper

¼ cup (15 g) finely chopped parsley

4 leaves Bibb lettuce, for serving

1 ripe tomato, quartered

Yield: 4 servings

Whisk together the mustard, lemon juice, and olive oil in a small bowl. Add the carrots, and season with salt and pepper to taste. Toss in parsley and mix well.

Serve garnished with Bibb lettuce and tomato wedges.

Mediterranean Tradition
Sometimes a variety of simple, already-assembled salads like this one are displayed beautifully at salad bars in restaurants in the region. Instead of making their own salads, as we do in the United States, patrons of the salad bar select from a dazzling array of salads already created for them. I adapted this style to my home kitchen where I often make up salads (without the dressings) in advance, store them in airtight containers, and enjoy a scoop of each for a quick and nutritious lunch or dinner.

Cream of Asparagus Soup/*Crema de Esparragos*

Asparagus soup is a classic first course in Spain. Served in clear glasses or little mugs, it makes a delicious and elegant starter. This soup is simple to make, and it reheats well.

2 pounds (910 g) asparagus, cleaned and trimmed

2 cups (475 ml) whole milk

2 cups (475 ml) water

¼ teaspoon unrefined sea salt or salt

Freshly ground pepper, to taste

4 tablespoons (16 g) parsley, finely chopped

Yield: 4 servings

Place the asparagus, milk, and water in a large saucepan. Add salt and pepper, and stir. Bring to a boil over high heat. Stir, reduce heat to medium-low, and simmer, uncovered, for 8 to 10 minutes, or until asparagus is tender.

Pour the soup into a blender. Remove the center spout from the lid to prevent it from bursting. Place the lid on the blender, and hold a kitchen towel over the center hole. Purée soup until it is blended. Whip the soup for 1 minute more and return it to the saucepan.

Heat the soup on low until warm. Taste and adjust seasonings, if necessary. Pour into clear glasses or coffee mugs, and top with parsley.

Mediterranean Tradition
When asparagus is bountiful during the spring in the northern Mediterranean region, it is transformed into a multitude of delicious dishes. Asparagus is packed with vitamins and minerals, which prevent many forms of cancer and heart disease.

Spaghetti Squash "Pasta" with Zucchini, Basil, and Cherry Tomatoes/*Spaghetti di zucca con zucchini, basilico e pomidori pacchini*

While spaghetti squash is hardly a grain, its tender strands do resemble golden noodles. Dressing it like pasta enhances its naturally sweet taste and transforms a simple side dish into a shining star on the table.

1 spaghetti squash (about 3½ pounds or 1.5 kg), halved and seeded

¼ cup (60 ml) extra-virgin olive oil, divided

1½ pints (345 g) cherry or grape tomatoes, halved

1 pound (455 g) zucchini, quartered, and cut into ¾-inch (2 cm) pieces

4 cloves garlic, minced

Unrefined sea salt or salt

Freshly ground pepper

6 fresh basil leaves, finely chopped

Grated Pecorino Romano cheese

Yield: 4 servings

Preheat the oven to 425°F (220°C).

Line a 15 x 10 x ½-inch (38 x 26 x 1 cm) baking pan with aluminum foil. Brush the cut surface of the squash with 1 tablespoon (15 ml) of oil; place it flesh-side down on the foil-lined pan. Roast on bottom rack 40 minutes, or until you can easily pierce the squash shell. When cool enough to handle, scrape the strands of spaghetti squash into a large bowl.

Place the tomatoes, zucchini, garlic, and remaining 3 tablespoons (45 ml) of oil in a 13 x 9-inch (33 x 23 cm) baking dish. Roast on the top rack for 30 minutes, or until tender.

Toss the zucchini, roasted tomatoes, and garlic. Season with salt and pepper, and stir in the basil. Spoon over the spaghetti squash. Sprinkle with Pecorino Romano.

Mediterranean Tradition
Spaghetti squash can be cut into cubes and roasted with olive oil, salt, and pepper, for a simple, sweet, and delicious side.

Roasted Red Pepper and Tomato Soup/
Shorbat tamatum bil filfil hamra

This soup is garnished with za'atar croutons and goat cheese. Try serving it in clear, heatproof cylindrical glasses for a stylish presentation. This soup can be made ahead of time and stored in the refrigerator. Reheat on low so that cream doesn't curdle. I always like to make extra croutons to eat with hummus and in salads.

For the Soup:

1 jar (12 ounce, or 340 g) fire-roasted peppers, drained

4 cups (950 ml) Chicken or Vegetable Stock (see page 183)

1 cup (180 g) chopped tomatoes

2 cloves garlic, chopped

Unrefined sea salt or salt, to taste

Freshly ground pepper, to taste

¼ cup (60 g) plain Greek yogurt

For the Za'atar Croutons:

1 pita, or any gluten-free bread, cut into 1-inch (2.5 cm) pieces

4 tablespoons (60 ml) olive oil

¼ cup (24 g) za'atar

6 teaspoons (6 g) goat cheese, for garnish

Yield: 4 to 6 servings

To make the soup: Combine the peppers, stock, tomatoes, garlic, salt, and freshly ground pepper in a medium saucepan. Bring to a boil over high heat and stir to mix well. Reduce heat to low, cover, and simmer for 20 minutes.

Remove from heat, stir, and pour into blender. Remove the spout on the lid and cover with a folded kitchen towel. Purée in blender until smooth and pour back into the saucepan. Stir in the yogurt and keep warm, on low, until ready to serve. Taste and adjust salt if necessary.

To make the croutons: Preheat the broiler. Brush olive oil onto the pita pieces and place on a baking sheet. Top with za'atar. Place under the broiler and toast until golden, 1 to 2 minutes on each side.

Pour the soup into serving cups or bowls. Top with za'atar croutons and a piece of goat cheese. Serve hot.

Mediterranean Tradition

Za'atar, which is made predominately from a variety of wild thyme, is used to cure coughs and bronchial illnesses in the eastern Mediterranean countries. Combined with olive oil and used as a dip for bread, it is the go-to remedy of many mothers. Many people might be surprised to learn that many modern cough syrups contain thymol, a natural derivative found in the oil of thyme, as an active ingredient.

Carrot, Coriander, and Parsnip Soup/*Soupe des carottes au coriandre avec les panais*

This sweet, creamy, sunset-colored soup never fails to impress guests. Best of all, it's easy to make, and good for you.

3 tablespoons (45 ml) extra-virgin olive oil

8 large carrots, peeled and sliced

2 parsnips, peeled and sliced

4 shallots, minced

1 teaspoon ground coriander

1 teaspoon unrefined sea salt or salt

Freshly ground black pepper

4 cups (950 ml) homemade or store-bought low-sodium Chicken Stock (see page 183)

¾ cup (175 ml) milk

¼ cup (4 g) finely chopped fresh cilantro

Yield: 4 to 6 servings

Heat the olive oil in a large saucepan with a lid. Add the carrots, parsnips, shallots, coriander, salt, and a pinch of pepper to the pot. Stir to combine. Reduce heat to medium-low, and sauté until tender, about 10 minutes.

Add the stock and milk, increase heat to high, and bring to a boil. Stir, reduce heat to medium-low and simmer for 20 minutes, or until the vegetables are tender.

Working in batches, carefully transfer to the jar of a blender (do not fill more than halfway). Remove center spout from lid to prevent it from bursting. Place lid on the blender, and hold a kitchen towel over the center hole. Purée the soup until it is blended and very smooth. Pour the soup back into saucepan and heat over low until warm. Taste and adjust seasonings. Serve in soup bowls garnished with cilantro.

Mediterranean Tradition
Carrots, packed with iron and beta carotene, are a wonderful addition to the diet. Fresh cilantro, and its dried counterpart, coriander, have been proven to regulate blood sugar levels in people with type II diabetes. All over the Mediterranean region, fresh grated carrots are often paired with cilantro in salads, and cooked carrots and coriander can be transformed into purées to serve alongside lean meats and poultry instead of mashed potatoes.

Sicilian Sweet and Sour Vegetable Medley/*Caponata*

This classic sweet and sour eggplant dish is rich and sweetened with caramelized onions and raisins. While the addition of chocolate may seem unorthodox to some, the Sicilian town of Modica—a UNESCO world heritage site—is actually famous for their chocolate, which is an ancient Aztec recipe introduced to Sicily by the Spaniards.

½ cup (120 ml) olive oil

1 eggplant (¾ pound, or 340 g), cut into 1-inch (2.5 cm) cubes

¼ yellow onion, finely chopped

⅓ rib celery, roughly chopped

kosher salt, to taste

Freshly ground black pepper, to taste

1 tablespoon (16 g) tomato paste, thinned with ¼ cup (60 ml) water

⅓ cup (76 g) canned crushed tomatoes

2 ounces (55 g) green olives, pitted and roughly chopped

2 tablespoons (30 ml) white wine vinegar

2 tablespoons (18 g) golden raisins

2 tablespoons (17 g) salt-packed capers, rinsed and drained

1 tablespoon (13 g) sugar

1 tablespoon (8 g) finely grated unsweetened chocolate

2 tablespoons (5 g) finely shredded basil

½ teaspoon pine nuts

4 pieces thinly sliced Italian bread, or gluten-free bread, rubbed with olive oil, and grilled or toasted on either side

Yield: 4 servings

Heat the oil in a 12-inch (30 cm) skillet over medium-high heat. Working in batches if necessary, add the eggplant and fry, tossing occasionally, until browned, 3 to 4 minutes. Using a slotted spoon, transfer the eggplant to a large paper towel–lined platter.

Add the onion and celery to the skillet, and season with salt and pepper. Cook, stirring often, until beginning to brown, 10 minutes. Reduce heat to medium, add tomato paste and cook, stirring, until caramelized and almost evaporated, 1 to 2 minutes.

Add the crushed tomatoes and continue cooking for 10 minutes. Stir in the olives, vinegar, raisins, capers, sugar, and chocolate, and cook, stirring occasionally, until thickened, about 15 minutes.

Transfer to a large bowl, then add the eggplant, along with basil and pine nuts, and mix together.

Season with salt and pepper, and let cool to room temperature before serving over toasted bread.

Mediterranean Tradition

All around the Mediterranean, people have been taking pride in procuring the best ingredients possible for their kitchens. Instead of hurried trips to the grocery store, families plan weekend outings to orchards, monasteries, marinas, and festivals known for their products. The excursions not only help to secure great ingredients but they also enhance family time and help preserve traditional foodways.

Braised Fennel with Chestnuts and Shallots/*Finocchio in padella con castagne e scalogni*

All across the Mediterranean region, fennel is celebrated for its mildly sweet flavor, culinary versatility, nutritional benefits, and budget-friendly price. Fennel is an herbaceous plant that originated in the Mediterranean region, where it has been used since 3000 BCE. The ancient Romans used dried fennel seeds to preserve foods. Fennel bulbs can be eaten raw, pickled, or cooked. The fennel stalks, which resemble celery, can be added into slow simmering stocks or stews for additional flavor.

2 tablespoons (30 ml) extra-virgin olive oil

3 large shallots, minced

3 pounds (1.4 kg) fennel, bulbs trimmed and quartered, a handful of fronds finely chopped and stalks reserved for another use

1 cup (235 ml) Vegetable Stock (see page 183)

½ teaspoon unrefined sea salt or salt

½ teaspoon freshly ground black pepper

1 package (5.28-ounces, or 150 g) roasted, shelled chestnuts

½ cup (30 g) freshly chopped Italian parsley

Yield: 6 servings

Heat the oil in a large skillet over medium heat. Add the shallots and sauté until translucent, 3 to 5 minutes. Add the fennel bulbs and cook for 5 minutes on each side, or until golden. Stir in the stock, salt, and pepper. Increase heat to high and bring to a boil. Stir in the chestnuts.

Reduce heat to low, cover, and simmer for 10 or 20 minutes, or until the fennel is tender and most of the liquid has reduced. Stir in the parsley, garnish with fronds, and serve warm.

Mediterranean Tradition
In the Mediterranean region, many people munch on raw fennel the way Americans may enjoy crunchy celery sticks. A single cup of fennel is a significant source of vitamin C and potassium.

Green Beans, Potatoes, and Cherry Tomatoes with Pesto/
Fagioli con patate e pomodori pacchini al pesto

Bright, basil-flavored pesto has enough flavor to perk up even the most boring vegetables. Pairing it with green beans, potatoes, and cherry tomatoes, however, is another story! This mixture is traditionally tossed into small, irregular shaped twisted pastas called *trofie* in the Liguria region of Italy, from which pesto hails. This dish is an excellent accompaniment to grilled or roasted fish, poultry, or meat.

1½ pounds (680 g) baby yellow potatoes or Yukon gold, washed and cut into 1-inch (2.5 cm) chunks

1 pound (455 g) green beans, trimmed and cut in half on the diagonal

1 cup (149 g) cherry tomatoes

¼ cup (35 g) pine nuts

1 clove garlic

3 cups (120 g) lightly packed fresh basil leaves

¼ cup (60 ml) extra-virgin olive oil, unfiltered if possible

¼ cup (25 g) freshly grated Parmigiano-Reggiano

Unrefined sea salt or salt

Freshly ground black pepper

Yield: 4 servings

Place the potatoes in a large steamer basket fitted over a pot of boiling water. Cover and steam for 5 minutes. Add the green beans to the potatoes in the steamer and continue to steam, covered, for another 4 minutes. Drain and immediately plunge into an ice bath to cool.

Make the pesto by combining the pine nuts, garlic, basil, and olive oil in a food processor. Process until a smooth paste forms. Using a spatula, scoop pesto out of food processor and into a bowl. Stir in cheese.

Transfer the vegetables to a large serving bowl and add cherry tomatoes. Add the pesto and stir to coat evenly. Season with salt and pepper to taste and serve.

Mediterranean Tradition
Unfiltered olive oil is often called raw olive oil. It contains microscopic particles of the olive which sink to the bottom of the bottle, and add more flavor and health benefits. Unfiltered olive oil shouldn't be heated, but rather consumed cold on salads, and in uncooked recipes such as pesto.

Moroccan Vegetable Tajine/*Tajine Khodhra*

Tajines are dishes named after the vessel in which they are cooked. A tajin (with emphasis on the first syllable) is the word for a clay pot in Arabic. In Morocco the word is pronounced *tajine* (with emphasis on the second syllable) and refers to a particular clay pot with a cone shaped lid that dishes are baked in. Seven is considered to be a lucky number in the Moroccan culture, so seven vegetables are used in this dish. This recipe is strictly vegetarian, though it is much more common to include meat in tajines in Morocco.

5 teaspoons (25 ml) extra-virgin olive oil, divided

2 yellow onions, finely chopped

¾ teaspoon unrefined sea salt or salt, divided

Freshly ground black pepper, to taste

1 teaspoon Ras el Hanout spice mixture

2 cups (475 ml) Vegetable or Chicken Stock (see page 183), boiling

1 pound (455 g) carrots, peeled and chopped into 1-inch (2.5 cm) pieces

½ pound (225 g) cauliflower florets

½ pound (225 g) frozen or canned artichoke hearts

½ pound (225 g) zucchini, chopped into 1-inch (2.5 cm) pieces

½ pound (225 g) eggplant, chopped into 1-inch (2.5 cm) pieces

½ pound (225 g) potatoes, peeled and cut into large chunks

½ pound (225 g) sweet potatoes, peeled and cut into large chunks

1 cup (175 g) couscous

Yield: 8 servings

Heat 1 teaspoon of olive oil in a large, heavy pot over medium heat. Add the onions and sauté until translucent, about 5 minutes. Add ¼ teaspoon salt, pepper, and Ras el Hanout spice mixture. Stir to combine. Pour in boiling vegetable or chicken stock and stir.

Add the carrots, cauliflower, artichoke hearts, zucchini, eggplant, potatoes, and sweet potatoes, and pour in enough water to cover three-quarters of the vegetables, and stir. Increase heat to high and bring to a boil, uncovered. Reduce heat to medium-low, and simmer for 45 minutes, until vegetables are very tender and have broken down.

Ten minutes before the tajine is finished, begin making couscous. Bring 3 cups (710 ml) water, 3 teaspoons (15 ml) of olive oil and remaining ½ teaspoon salt to a boil in a medium saucepan over high heat. Take the saucepan off heat, add couscous, stir, and cover with a lid.

Let stand for ten minutes. Remove lid, fluff with fork, and stir in remaining teaspoon of olive oil. Serve in a large, shallow dish next to the tajine. When the tajine is finished, serve warm with ½ cup (88 g) of couscous per serving.

Mediterranean Tradition
Clay pot cooking is extremely healthful because it seals the nutrients in the stew, and it requires very little cooking oil to produce a great deal of flavor. Each country in the region—from France to Egypt—has their own version.

Mixed Greens with Grapes, Goat Cheese, and Herbs/ *Insalata mista con l'uva, formaggio di capra ed erbe*

This salad makes a great first course, and an impressive addition to any pot luck. The combination of grapes, goat cheese, and herbs are divine, and the orange blossom water–infused vinaigrette brings this salad to life!

1 head romaine lettuce

1 cup (150 g) red seedless grapes

½ cup (48 g) finely chopped fresh mint

½ cup (30 g) finely chopped fresh parsley

¼ cup (60 ml) extra-virgin olive oil

Juice of 1 orange

1 teaspoon orange blossom water

Unrefined sea salt or salt

Freshly ground black pepper

1 cup (150 g) goat cheese

Yield: 4 servings

Chop the lettuce into bite-size pieces and place in a large bowl or serving platter. Toss in grapes, mint, and parsley, and set aside. Make the dressing by pouring olive oil into a small bowl. Whisk in orange juice and orange blossom water, and season with salt and pepper to taste.

Using a melon baller or teaspoons, shape the goat cheese into equal-size balls. Arrange cheese on top of salad. Drizzle dressing over the top. Season with salt and freshly ground black pepper, to taste.

Mediterranean Tradition
The tradition of serving goat cheese with herbs dates back to antiquity when farmers would decorate the edges of goat cheese wheels with the same herbs that the goats who produced the milk to make the cheese grazed on. That way, a consumer could tell which flavor the cheese would have. While many vendors simply decorate modern goat cheese with herbs for ornamental reasons, the flavors still taste great together and provide nutrients and visual interest to any meal. Look for the freshest variety possible.

Lebanese Fattoush Salad/*Salata Fattoush*

Originally from the eastern Mediterranean countries of Lebanon and Syria, fattoush salad is a delicious cucumber and tomato salad tossed with crunchy toasted pita pieces and dressed with pomegranate molasses and sumac dressing. Mediterranean sumac, different from the American variety, is obtained by grinding the seeds of the sumac plant, which is a member of the cashew family. It produces a beautiful red powder that gives a tangy taste to chicken, eggs, spice mixes, rice, and dips. Look for it at Mediterranean markets.

1 cucumber, diced

4 Roma tomatoes, finely chopped

1 medium red onion, thinly sliced

1 green pepper, seeded and diced

1 Whole-Wheat Pita Bread (page 19), or gluten-free bread, cut into 12 pieces

2 teaspoons sumac

2 tablespoons (30 ml) extra-virgin olive oil

1 tablespoon (20 g) pomegranate molasses

Juice of 1 lemon (about ¼ cup, or 60 ml)

1 teaspoon white wine vinegar

½ teaspoon dried mint

¼ teaspoon kosher salt

¼ teaspoon freshly ground pepper, to taste

Yield: 8 servings

Combine the cucumber, tomatoes, red onion, and green pepper in a large salad bowl.

Preheat the broiler. Sprinkle the pita pieces with sumac, and place under the broiler and toast for 2 to 4 minutes, until golden on both sides. Remove the pita from oven and set aside to cool.

Mix olive oil, pomegranate molasses, lemon juice, white wine vinegar, mint, salt, and pepper in a medium bowl. Whisk vigorously to form a smooth dressing.

Add the pita chips to the salad and toss to combine. Pour the dressing over salad and toss again to combine. Serve immediately.

Mediterranean Tradition
Toss leftover morsels of meat or chicken, or cooked beans, lentils, or quinoa with Fattoush Salad for a quick lunch or dinner.

LEGUMES AND NUTS

Lentil soup. Hummus. Falafel. Some of the first dishes that come to mind when we think about Mediterranean cuisine include legumes. Perhaps it's because many legume-based recipes have been around in the Mediterranean since antiquity: Fava beans are actually the world's oldest agricultural crop, whereas wild chickpeas were first cultivated 11,000 years ago! Luckily for us, many heirloom beans and lentils, packed with nutrients and protein, are readily available and inexpensive today.

Legumes and nuts are to a cook what a blank canvas is to an artist. Mild in flavor and easy to prepare, there are thousands of ways to transform the tiny little beans and lentils into extraordinary dishes. Often dismissed as *cucina povera,* or poor man's food, beans and lentils are often overlooked when planning elegant menus. It's important to note, however, that beans and especially lentils were worth their weight in gold in various times in history. For that reason, they are often eaten at New Year's in Italy, in order to ensure a prosperous new year.

Nuts are much more than just a snack or party food in the Mediterranean region. They're actually a celebrated ingredient—often incorporated into fillings, dips, and sauces—and play center stage in pastry making. Pistachios, almonds, walnuts, and pine nuts are the most popular throughout the region, along with peanuts in Egypt. Toasted and fried nuts with raisins make a sweet, crunchy garnish for sautéed spinach and rice dishes. Increasing your legume and nut repertoire provides great health benefits and can heighten your cooking skills.

Nutritional Benefits

Beans and legumes provide the main sources of daily protein in the Mediterranean diet. Rich in fiber, they can help to slow down digestion and prevent huge swings in blood sugar—a major plus for diabetics. Legumes and nuts contain large amounts of vitamins B_{12} and B_6, protein, iron, magnesium, zinc, thiamin, niacin, phosphorus, and magnesium. Beans are similar to animal proteins in that they are a good source of protein, but unlike the animal proteins, they are fat free. It is important to note that a little goes a long way when it comes to legumes. Serving sizes of legumes and nuts differ from animal sources. Only ¼ cup (55 g) of cooked beans is considered a full serving. Most healthy adults should consume 5 to 7 ounces (140 to 195 g) of protein foods per day.

Nuts are often avoided by health-conscious individuals because of their high caloric content. Remember, though, that since they are high in heart-healthy monounsaturated fat, the quality of calories that they provide is very high, making them an extremely satisfying food.

They also contain high amounts of copper, magnesium, protein, fiber, selenium, vitamin E, and antioxidants. Various studies have shown that people, including those who were already following a Mediterranean diet, were able to decrease their LDL (bad) cholesterol and total cholesterol simply by increasing the amounts of pistachios, almonds, and walnuts they ate. In fact, adding 3 ounces (85 g) of almonds to the daily diet was shown to drop total cholesterol by 9 percent in just nine weeks.

"Growing up in the country, where we produced high-quality beans, I have developed a finicky appreciation for good, fresh beans. Basilicata is, in fact, famous for its beans; we even have festivals, or sagre, in their honor. In ancient times, beans and legumes were used as a form of currency. Later, when the rich turned to a meat-heavy diet, beans and legumes became the 'meat of the poor.' With their proven health benefits, however, I believe they are set to make a strong comeback on the culinary scene. As the Slow Food Organization states, beans, favas, chickpeas, lentils, and the like are the foods of the future."

—*Chef Luigi Diotaiuti*

Herb-Infused Falafel/*Falafel*

Falafel's popularity in the Middle East dates back to antiquity. This is the eastern Mediterranean version, which can be found everywhere from Israel to Lebanon, Syria, and Turkey. In Egypt, the same recipe is prepared with dried fava beans instead of chickpeas. Note that the chickpeas used in this recipe need to be soaked overnight, and the falafel mixture needs to rest for a minimum of 1 hour before frying.

1 cup (171 g) dried chickpeas, soaked overnight in water and drained

¼ cup (6 g) fresh mint

¼ cup (4 g) fresh cilantro

¼ cup (15 g) fresh parsley

1 small yellow onion, diced

8 cloves garlic, chopped

1 teaspoon ground cumin

1 teaspoon ground coriander

Pinch of cayenne pepper

Unrefined sea salt or salt

Freshly ground black pepper

1 teaspoon baking powder

Expeller pressed canola or corn oil, for frying

¼ cup (36 g) white sesame seeds

4 loaves Whole-Wheat Pita Bread (see page 19)

2 Roma tomatoes, thinly sliced

1 cucumber, thinly sliced

¼ pound (115 g) feta cheese, crumbled

Tahini Sauce:

¼ cup (57 g) tahini

1 clove garlic, mashed

1 teaspoon lemon juice

1 teaspoon vinegar

Dash of cayenne

¼ teaspoon salt

Yield: 4 to 6 servings

Place the chickpeas in a saucepan covered with water. Bring to a boil over high heat, reduce heat to low, cover, and simmer for about 1 hour, or until tender. Drain.

Place the chickpeas, mint, cilantro, parsley, onion, and garlic into a food processor and mix until a smooth paste forms. Mix in ½ cup (120 ml) water or enough to make mixture wet and loose—it should resemble the thickness of a thin paste. Add the cumin, coriander, cayenne, salt, and pepper. Stir in the baking powder and mix to incorporate. Spoon the mixture into a bowl and let stand at room temperature for 1 hour.

Pour 3 inches (7.5 cm) of oil in a large frying pan over medium heat. The oil is hot enough to fry when a piece of bread dropped in will turn golden and float to the top. Using two teaspoons, gather the paste in one spoon and carefully push it off with the other spoon, forming a round patty, into the oil. While the falafel is frying, sprinkle a few sesame seeds on the uncooked side. Repeat the process until the pan is full, leaving a ½-inch (1.3 cm) space between each falafel. Fry until dark golden brown, about 5 minutes, turn over, and fry the other side until it is the same color.

Line a platter with paper towels. Using a slotted spoon, lift the falafel out of oil and drain on a plate lined with paper towels. Repeat with remaining dough. Serve warm in halved pieces of pita with tomatoes, cucumber, cheese, and tahini sauce.

To make the tahini sauce: Combine the tahini, garlic, lemon juice, and vinegar together in a medium bowl, mixing well. Add water, one tablespoon at a time, to thin the sauce to a syrupy consistency. Stir in cayenne. Cover and store in refrigerator until needed.

Mediterranean Tradition

Tahini is a sesame paste made from pressing the oil from sesame seeds. The attractive flowers of the tropical sesame plant produce sesame seeds as they dry up. They yield approximately a tablespoon (3 g) per pod. Since sesame plants grown in abundance in the Southern United States, its cost remains relatively low considering its array of healthful properties.

Chickpea Salad/*Nohut Piyazi*

This light yet filling Turkish salad is adapted from *A Taste of Turkish Cuisine* by Nur Ilkin and Sheilah Kaufman. Sheilah is my cookbook mentor and has written twenty-six cookbooks in addition to this and another with Nur Ilkin, wife of the former Ambassador of Turkey to the United States.

For the Chickpeas:
15 ounces (425 g) cooked chickpeas (page 182), or 1 can chickpeas, rinsed and drained

1 medium red onion, finely chopped

½ green bell pepper, seeded, ribbed, and finely chopped

½ bunch Italian parsley, washed, dried, and finely chopped

Dressing:
Juice of 1 lemon

2 teaspoons white vinegar

½ teaspoon unrefined sea salt or salt

½ teaspoon sugar

½ cup (120 ml) extra-virgin olive oil

Garnish:
2 hard cooked eggs, quartered

Yield: 4 servings

To make the salad: Place the chickpeas in a large bowl and add onions, bell peppers, and parsley. Mix well.

To make the dressing: In a small bowl, whisk together the lemon juice, vinegar, salt, sugar, and oil.

To garnish and serve: Pour dressing over the chickpea mixture and toss to mix and combine. Garnish with the egg slices and serve.

Mediterranean Tradition
It's no wonder chickpeas are so popular in the Mediterranean. Two cups (328 g) a day provides the entire recommended daily requirement of fiber. They also grow abundantly and are inexpensive. Eaten in salads, stews, soups, dips, and roasted as snacks, there's no reason why they can't be enjoyed every day.

Silky Hummus with Yogurt and Pomegranate Seeds/
Hummus bil tahini wa zabadi

If you are a fan of traditional hummus, you'll love this extra creamy version studded with pretty, ruby-colored pomegranate seeds. You can make large quantities of this hummus and store it in an airtight container in the refrigerator for up to a week.

2 cups (480 g) cooked or no-salt-added canned chickpeas (see page 182)

1 clove garlic, minced

⅓ cup (80 g) tahini (sesame purée)

2 teaspoons extra-virgin olive oil, plus extra for drizzling

½ teaspoon unrefined sea salt or salt

½ cup (115 g) plain Greek or plain, full-fat yogurt

Handful of pomegranate seeds

Yield: 4 servings

Place the chickpeas in a food processor, reserving a few for garnish. Add the garlic, tahini, olive oil, and salt to the food processor. Purée until smooth.

Add water, tablespoon by tablespoon, to get a creamy consistency. You should need less than ¼ cup (60 ml) in total. Scrape down the sides of the food processor, add the yogurt, and purée for 1 to 2 additional minutes. Taste and adjust salt if necessary.

Scoop the hummus onto a medium-size plate. Smooth out the top and make a dent in the middle. Drizzle with olive oil and sprinkle pomegranate seeds over the top.

Mediterranean Tradition
Serve dips and purées with raw vegetable crudités instead of bread for a more nutritious snack or appetizer.

Pomegranate, Roasted Red Pepper, and Walnut Dip/ *Muhammara*

This piquant, sweet and sour dip has origins in Persia and is now popular across the Middle East and in Turkey. Recently touted as a "beauty dip" by American magazines for the skin enhancing qualities found in its three main ingredients—red peppers, walnuts, and pomegranate—this recipe is quick to become a favorite of those who try it for the first time.

1 jar (7 ounces, or 198 g) roasted red peppers, drained and rinsed

⅓ cup (17 g) Fresh Bread Crumbs (see page 182), or almond flour

⅓ cup (27 g) walnuts

4 cloves garlic, minced

Juice of 1 lemon

4 tablespoons (80 g) pomegranate molasses

Pinch of cayenne pepper

Unrefined sea salt or salt

¼ cup (60 ml) extra-virgin olive oil

Yield: 4 servings

Combine the peppers, bread crumbs, walnuts, garlic cloves, lemon juice, pomegranate molasses, cayenne pepper, and salt in a food processor. Pulse on and off until a thick paste forms. Then, gradually pour olive oil into the running food processor. Taste the purée and adjust the salt as needed. Serve at room temperature.

Mediterranean Tradition
Pomegranates were present in 1550 BCE in Egypt and begin appearing in Greek mythology three thousand years ago. Throughout history, their juice and seeds were used in natural medicines for curing a wide variety of ailments. Pomegranates made their way to Spain and were introduced to America with Spanish settlers in 1769. They are now grown in California and Arizona. Modern doctors have been researching the fruit and found that it helps reduce the risk of heart disease and colon cancer, and can also lower high blood pressure. It also helps to inhibit the spread of other cancers.

Fava Beans with Chicory/*Fave con cicorie*

This recipe is from *The Al Tiramisu Restaurant Cookbook* by Luigi Diotaiuti, who says, "Natives of Puglia in southern Italy proudly associate this dish with their culinary patrimony. But it's also popular in parts of my region, which shares a border with Puglia. Recipes for this dish can vary—almost from one household to another. Fava beans, one of the world's oldest agricultural crops, have long been a staple of southern Italian cooking. But thanks to Queen Margherita, wife of King Umberto of the Kingdom of Italy in the late 1800s, this dish and other 'street food' was introduced to Italian nobility and eventually the rest of the world. Serve this dish alone or as part of a mixed appetizer platter." Note that the fava beans must be soaked overnight.

11 ounces (312 g) dried peeled fava beans, placed in a bowl, covered with boiling water (4 inches [10 cm]) above top of beans), and left to soak overnight

½ small onion

4 ounces (115 g) potatoes, diced

1 teaspoon unrefined sea salt or salt

7 ounces (198 g) chicory or dandelion greens, cleaned

⅓ cup (80 ml) good-quality olive oil, preferably from Puglia, divided

2 cloves garlic, thinly sliced

Yield: 4 servings

Drain the soaked fava beans and place them in a medium saucepan.

Add the onion, potato, and salt. Cover with water and bring to a boil over high heat. Reduce heat to medium-low, cover, and cook until beans are tender, about 25 minutes. This could take longer depending on the size of the beans.

In a medium saucepan, cook the chicory or dandelion greens in enough salted boiling water to cover for 2 minutes. Drain and reserve the cooking liquid.

Transfer the beans and vegetables to a food processor or food mill. Purée until smooth, adding a tablespoon (15 ml) of the olive oil and additional salt, if needed. Add a few tablespoons of the reserved cooking water, if needed. Heat a tablespoon (15 ml) of olive oil in a medium skillet over medium heat. Add the garlic and cook until it turns golden, about 1 minute. Add the chicory or dandelion greens. Stir well and cook for a couple minutes, to absorb flavors. Season with salt to taste.

To serve, spread the fava purée in the bottom of a terra-cotta bowl. Mound the chicory in the center. Drizzle the remaining olive oil on top and serve.

Mediterranean Tradition
It's said that there are 60 million olive trees in Puglia—one for every Italian. A drizzle of great Puglia olive oil brings this humble dish to life. Do as the Italians do: Use a basic first cold-pressed, extra-virgin olive oil for cooking. Then, buy the best quality unfiltered olive oil to drizzle on top of dishes such as this one.

Egyptian Cream of Lentil Soup/*Shorbat Ads*

I've always loved lentil soups in all their guises—but in my opinion, the Egyptians make them best. During ancient times, Egyptians were the chief exporters of lentils in the world. Since lentils were traded for currency, and their shape is reminiscent of small coins, they are often associated with wealth. I like to serve lentils on New Year's Eve to wish my guests, and myself, a prosperous, healthy, new year.

2 teaspoons olive oil

1 onion, diced

2 carrots, diced

2 ribs celery, diced

1 cup (192 g) brown lentils, rinsed

1 teaspoon ground coriander

Unrefined sea salt or salt

Freshly ground black pepper

4 cups (940 g) Vegetable or Chicken Stock (see page 183)

Croutons, for garnish

Yield: 4 servings

Heat the oil in a large saucepan over medium heat. Add the onion, carrots, and celery. Sauté until translucent (3 to 5 minutes), stir, and add lentils. Cook for 1 minute, add the coriander and season with salt and freshly ground pepper to taste. Add the stock, stir, and increase heat to high.

When the stock begins to boil, reduce heat to medium-low and stir. Cover and allow to simmer for 30 to 45 minutes, or until lentils are tender. Taste and adjust salt and pepper if necessary. Blend with an immersion blender or in blender and serve warm with croutons.

Mediterranean Tradition
Try swapping out other beans or legumes for variety in this delicious, hearty soup. You can make large batches of the soup and freeze it in individual portions for a quick and nutritious lunch anytime.

Chickpea Soup with Shrimp/
Crema di ceci con gamberi

The combination of homemade stock, chickpeas, and shrimp with herbs make this soup sing! Chickpeas are a good source of protein, calcium, phosphorus, potassium, and magnesium. Consider adding them to salads, soups, pastas, rice, and couscous dishes the way people in the Mediterranean region do to take advantage of their health benefits.

For the Stock:
½ pound (225 g) shrimp, peels reserved and deveined

1 carrot

1 onion, peeled and halved

1 rib celery

Unrefined sea salt or salt

5 black peppercorns or ¼ teaspoon ground black pepper

1 bay leaf

For the Chickpea Soup:
1 cup (171 g) dried chickpeas, soaked overnight, rinsed, and drained well, or 1 can (15 ounces, or 425 g), drained and rinsed

1 lemon, juiced

For the Shrimp:
Unrefined sea salt or salt, to taste

Freshly ground black pepper, to taste

1 tablespoon (15 ml) extra-virgin olive oil

½ teaspoon chopped fresh rosemary

Yield: 4 servings

To make the shrimp stock: (This step can be done 1 day ahead.) Place the shrimp peels in a large stockpot with 8 cups (2 L) water, carrot, onion, and celery. Bring to a boil over high heat. Skim scum off the top of the pot and carefully discard. Add 1 tablespoon (18 g) salt, peppercorns, and bay leaf. Reduce heat to medium-low and simmer for 30 minutes and strain.

To make the chickpea soup: Place the chickpeas in a large saucepan or stockpot with 6 cups (1.5 L) of shrimp stock and an onion. Simmer, covered, on medium-low until the chickpeas are tender (1 hour for dried chickpeas or about 5 minutes for canned).

Take off the heat and drain, reserving cooking liquid. Place the chickpeas and the reserved liquid in blender. Add lemon juice, and the salt, and pepper to taste. Blend well until a purée is formed.

Return the mixture to the pot. Taste, and adjust salt if necessary. If the soup is too thick, stir in a few tablespoons of water. Stir and simmer on low heat until ready to serve.

To make the shrimp: Heat the olive oil in a large skillet over medium-high heat. When the olive oil begins to release its aroma, add the shrimp and rosemary, and salt to taste. Cook for 1 to 2 minutes per side, or just until the shrimp lose their gray color, begin to turn bright pink and are cooked through.

Garnish soup with shrimp on top.

Note: If you don't have time to make homemade shrimp stock, you can substitute water or seafood stock in this recipe. You can also freeze the shrimp shells to make stock at a later time. The stock can also be made ahead of time and frozen in a plastic container for up to 1 month. To defrost, place in a bowl in the refrigerator for 24 hours.

Mediterranean Tradition
I highly recommend making your own stock for this recipe because it is delicious, easy, and a much more healthful alternative to sodium-laden, store-bought recipes. It also gives this recipe a light, clean taste.

Italian Pasta with Chickpeas/*Pasta con ceci*

Various types of pasta with chickpeas are famous throughout Italy. Chickpeas were once a symbol of rebirth in southern Italy and other areas of the Mediterranean. Local pastas such as cavatelli and lagane, which were prepared with whole-grain flour since the fourth century BCE in the region, were paired with chickpeas and served at harvest times. Cavatelli are small cave-shaped little shell-like pasta shapes ubiquitous to my ancestral homeland of Calabria, Italy, where the older generation of housewives still makes them by hand. The best ones I ever tasted were the ones my aunt Zia Santina used to make. Because cavatelli can be difficult to find outside of Southern Italy, you can substitute your short- or medium-grain pasta of choice with this recipe.

8 ounces (225 g) chickpeas, soaked in water to cover overnight and drained

1 bay leaf

1 clove garlic

3 teaspoons unrefined sea salt or salt, divided

4 tablespoons (60 ml) good-quality extra-virgin olive oil

1 onion, finely chopped

1 small chile pepper, finely chopped

¾ pound (340 g) cherry tomatoes, quartered

6 fresh basil leaves, shredded, or 1 tablespoon (4 g) finely chopped parsley

Freshly ground black pepper

1 pound (455 g) cavatelli, or any small, gluten-free pasta

Pecorino Crotonese or Pecorino Romano, for serving

Yield: 4 servings

Place the chickpeas, bay leaf, garlic clove, and 1 teaspoon salt in a large saucepan, cover with water, and bring to a boil over high heat. Reduce heat to low, and simmer, covered, adding hot water as needed, for 30 minutes. Drain and remove the bay leaf. This step can be done up to a week in advance.

In a large skillet, heat the olive oil over medium heat. Add the onion and sauté until soft, 3 to 5 minutes. Add the chile pepper, tomatoes, and basil or parsley. Stir in 1 teaspoon salt and black pepper, to taste. Allow to cook 5 minutes.

Add the cooked chickpeas to the tomato mixture, cover, and simmer for 30 minutes, or until chickpeas are tender.

Bring a large pot of water to boil over high heat. Season with a teaspoon of salt, add the cavatelli, stir, and reduce heat to medium-low. Allow to cook for about 10 minutes, or until pasta is al dente.

Drain the pasta and toss it with ladlefuls of the sauce. Garnish with freshly grated Pecorino and serve.

Mediterranean Tradition
Pairing quality, whole-grain pastas with legumes, vegetables, and cheese make great vegetarian meals in minutes.

Pomegranate, Lentil, and Mixed Green Salad/ *Salata khadra bi ruman wa ads*

This salad combines protein-packed lentils with sweet and tart pomegranate seeds and crunchy mixed greens for a sweet and savory combination that tastes as good as it is healthy.

½ cup (96 g) lentils, rinsed, drained, and sorted

1 bay leaf

4 cups (120 g) mixed field greens or baby spinach

¼ cup (45 g) pomegranate arils (seeds)

¼ cup (60 ml) pomegranate juice

2 tablespoons (30 ml) extra-virgin olive oil

Unrefined sea salt or salt, to taste

Freshly ground black pepper, to taste

Yield: 4 servings

Place the lentils in a medium saucepan and cover with water. Bring to a boil over high heat, reduce heat to low, and add the bay leaf. Simmer, uncovered, for 30 minutes, or until tender. Drain, and discard the bay leaf.

Divide the mixed greens evenly among 4 salad plates. Sprinkle pomegranate arils over the greens.

Heat the pomegranate juice in a small saucepan over medium-high heat until it boils. Reduce heat to low and simmer for 5 to 10 minutes, until thick and syrupy.

Slowly pour in the olive oil while whisking vigorously to form a homogenous dressing. Taste and season with salt and pepper as needed. Sprinkle lentils evenly over the salad and drizzle dressing over the top.

Mediterranean Tradition
Try preparing lentils in large batches in advance so that they will be on hand and can easily be incorporated into recipes when needed.

Moroccan Harira Soup/*Harira*

Harira is a traditional, hearty, Moroccan soup that is eaten as the sundown break-fast meal during the month of Ramadan. Harira tends to thicken as it stands. If making a day in advance, you may choose to add more water or stock to it before reheating it. This soup also freezes well.

2 tablespoons (30 ml) extra-virgin olive oil

1 pound (455 g) boneless beef, lamb, veal, or goat shoulder meat cubes (1 inch, or 2.5 cm)

1 medium yellow onion, diced

1 rib celery, finely chopped

½ cup (96 g) lentils, sorted, rinsed, and drained

½ cup (125 g) tomato purée

6 cups (1. 5 L) Chicken, Beef, or Vegetable Stock (see page 183), or water

1 teaspoon Ras el Hanout spice mix

½ teaspoon unrefined sea salt or salt

¼ cup (49 g) medium-grain rice

¼ cup (4 g) cilantro, roughly chopped

¼ cup (15 g) parsley, roughly chopped

1 cup (240 g) cooked chickpeas (see page 182)

1 tablespoon (16 g) tomato paste

Yield: 4 servings

Heat the oil in a large, heavy-bottomed saucepan over medium heat. Add the meat, onion, and celery, and stir to combine. Brown the meat and sauté the vegetables until soft, 3 to 5 minutes. Add the lentils, tomato purée, stock, Ras el Hanout, and salt. Bring to a boil over high heat, stir and reduce heat to low. Cover and simmer for an hour. The vegetables will be tender and the meat almost done.

Carefully remove the lid and add the rice, cilantro, parsley, chickpeas, and tomato paste to the pot. Stir, increase heat to high, and bring to a boil. Reduce heat to low, cover, and simmer for another 20 minutes, or until meat, vegetables, and rice are tender, and soup has thickened.

Mediterranean Tradition

Stretching soup with seasonal vegetables and grains is a traditional way of serving large groups in an inexpensive and healthy way. There is a traditional Calabrian proverb that says that soup does seven things: "It cures hunger, quenches your thirst, fills your stomach, cleans your teeth, makes you sleep, helps you digest, and puts color in your cheeks."

OLIVE OIL

Olives are the ingredient most commonly associated with the Mediterranean diet—and for good reason! There are more than 750 million olive trees in the region, comprising 95 percent of the world's total. It is said that 25 to 40 percent of the daily caloric intake of Mediterranean people comes from olive oil. Olive products are the common denominator that the cuisines of the entire region, from southern France to Israel, rely on. Further, olives, olive wood, olive oil, and its pumice are used to make everything from food and furniture to fuel and soap.

Olive harvest time has always been associated with good fortune and celebration. There is an Italian saying that says that grapes, grains, and olives make up the holy trinity of foods. First domesticated 8,000 years ago in the eastern Mediterranean areas that comprise modern day Israel, Syria, Palestine, and Lebanon, archeologists have found olive pits dating back 8,000 years and evidence of olive oil production from 6,000 years ago. By the fourth millennium BCE, the ancient Egyptians were using olive oil not only for culinary purposes, but also for cosmetics and perfumes. Since perfume making was so important to the Mediterranean at the time, the role of olive oil in its production made olives an important crop.

Often called *green gold*, or *liquid gold*, olive oil has a symbolic meaning in the three monotheistic faiths—Judaism, Christianity, and Islam. Hanukah commemorates the miracle of one day's worth of olive oil lasting eight nights as recorded in the Talmud. Christians use olive oil to consecrate crowned rulers and church dignitaries. The Qur'an mentions olives numerous times and the Prophet Muhammad is said to have proclaimed, "Take oil of olive and massage with it. It is a blessed tree."

Hippocrates prescribed olive oil for curing gastric ulcers, muscular pain, and cholera. In the southern Italian region of Calabria, where my family is from, a few drops are added into the water of a baby's first bath to ensure that he or she will have good skin for life. In many places in the Mediterranean region, it is rubbed into babies' gums to soothe teething pain. Spanish physicians discovered that it was more effective than quinine in treating malaria! In Tuscany, olive oil was considered to be "one of the four most necessary things in the life of man."

Whether drizzling over salads, dips, yogurt and cheese, using it to sauté vegetables or simmer sauces, deep frying, and even in dessert, olive oil can't be missed. It is best served fresh, but it can fortunately keep for a very long time without going rancid. Contrary to popular belief, it actually has a high smoke point, 365°F to 400°F (185°C to 200°C) depending on the type, which is why people in the region fry with it. To make sure it stays fresh for a longer period, always store olive oil away from light.

Types of Olive Oil

Olive oils are categorized by their acidity level and extraction method. There are both domestic and imported olive oils on the market that do not meet the standards of a true extra-virgin olive oil. One way to ensure quality when purchasing olive oil is to seek out varieties and brands that come from countries such as Italy, Greece, France, and Spain, which do regulate olive oil labels with government seals of approval. A harvest date printed on the label ensures freshness. Source of origin of olives is also important, although the phrase "packaged in" simply means that the olives weren't grown in that country, only bottled there. Here are further ways to decode the labels.

Single variety: Made from one variety of olives that may come from a single estate or growing area of a particular country or region instead of a more common commercial blend of olives.

Pure: The most inexpensive, made out of a combination of refined virgin and extra-virgin olive oils. Many people use this type of oil for frying.

Light: Refers to a lighter colored olive oil that has been filtered to remove the olive sediment, and may have a less "olivey" flavor. It does not refer to the fat or calories of the oil.

Virgin: Comes from the mechanical expeller of olives, contains 1–2% acid, and has not been refined or treated with heat. Along with extra-virgin, it has the largest amount of antioxidants.

Extra-virgin: Has the lowest amount of acidity (1%). It also comes from the first pressing of olives done with cold extraction. It has the freshest, most fruity flavor, and is considered to be the highest quality.

First cold-pressed: Oil is extracted from the first pressing of the olives, which denotes better quality and flavor. True extra-virgin olive oils are all first cold pressed.

Unfiltered: Contains small particles of olive flesh, which reduces shelf life of the oil. Many people, myself included, feel that unfiltered olive oil has greater taste because the olive particles continue to flavor it.

According to the International Olive Oil Council, to determine whether an olive oil is truly extra-virgin, "Place a small quantity of the oil in a glass bowl and refrigerate it for a few days. If it becomes crystalline, the chances are good that it is a true extra-virgin olive oil. If it forms a block, it is most likely chemically refined oil that has had some first-pressed oil added to it."

Nutritional Benefits

Because olives and olive oil are a common denominator in the countries surrounding the Mediterranean, they are often the ingredients that are analyzed in Mediterranean diet–based research.

Olives are rich in beta carotene, calcium, iron, dietary fiber, antioxidant nutrients (vitamins A and E, flavonoids, and polyphenols), and monounsaturated fatty acids. Monounsaturated fats have anti-inflammatory effects, which can help prevent heart disease, lower cholesterol, improve rheumatoid arthritis, and reduce the risk of developing Alzheimer's disease, diabetes, and various types of cancer. Further, various studies have shown that olive oil or an olive oil–rich diet:

- can protect against malignant tumors

- reduces the risk of breast, colon, and bowel cancer and the incidence of melanoma

- prevents the formation of blood clots and lowers the levels of total blood cholesterol (believed to be responsible for the low incidence of heart problems in countries where olive oil is the main cooking fat)

- boosts the immune system against the negative effects of toxins, microorganisms, parasites, and other foreign substances

- can improve calcium absorption in the body and prevent osteoporosis

- may prevent memory loss in healthy elderly people

- may lead to less risk of developing rheumatoid arthritis

Antioxidants such as vitamin E, carotenoids, and phenols (known for their anti-inflammatory and antibacterial effects) are found in olive oil. It's important to note, however, that the amount of antioxidants in olive oils varies according to the climate where the olives are raised, when the olives are harvested, how ripe they are when they are picked, and how the oil is produced and stored. Antioxidants are important in the prevention of aging. Oxidation refers to the complex manner in which cells age. Cells in those following olive oil–rich diets have been proven to be stronger and more resistant to oxidation, and therefore age more slowly. The Mediterranean diet's positive effect on longevity is accredited to its high antioxidant content. Virgin olive oil (olive oil that has not been refined or industrially treated) is particularly rich in antioxidants, which protects against damage from free radicals and against the formation of cancer.

The body's overall ease in digestion and absorption of olive oil, as well as the need for its many nutrients, make it an ideal cooking ingredient and traditional medicinal.

Kale and Almond Pesto Sauce/
Pesto di ravizzone e mandorle

This is a quick and delicious uncooked sauce, perfect for busy evenings that require something delicious and nutritious. I upped the nutrition factor on the traditional Basil Pesto by replacing the basil with kale and the pine nuts with almonds. The strong flavors work beautifully with healthful whole-wheat and gluten-free quinoa pastas while delivering extra vitamins and minerals. This recipe makes enough sauce for 1 pound (455 g) of pasta. I prefer short cuts such as fusilli and farfalle for this sauce.

¾ cup (175 ml) good-quality extra-virgin olive oil

3 cups (200 g) fresh baby kale

2 cloves garlic

¼ cup (36 g) whole almonds

¼ cup (25 g) freshly grated Parmigiano-Reggiano cheese

¼ cup (25 g) freshly grated Romano cheese

Yield: 6 servings (enough for 1 pound of pasta)

Place all of the ingredients except the cheese in a food processor. Mix to combine and form a smooth paste. Scoop the mixture out of food processor into a bowl. Stir in the cheese.

Mediterranean Tradition
Pesto sauce should never be heated. To freeze pesto, mix to combine all ingredients except the cheese, cover the top with additional olive oil, and place in an airtight container. Thaw overnight in the refrigerator before using. Pesto can also be stored in the refrigerator for up to 1 week.

Herb-Marinated Olives/*Olive marinate*

This is a standard recipe for marinating olives that can be changed to suit your taste. I began using it when my dear friend Rosa Vilella, a native of Valencia, Spain, used to bring me her freshly brined olives. Rosa was one of the best cooks I ever had the pleasure of knowing. Entering her home was like taking a trip to Spain. I try to include at least one of her recipes in each of my cookbooks in hopes that the memory of her beautiful spirit will live on through them.

4 cups (512 g) assorted brine-cured olives (such as kalamata, Gaeta, or Niçoise), rinsed, drained

1½ cups (360 ml) fine quality extra-virgin olive oil

6 fresh oregano sprigs

6 whole black peppercorns

4 large cloves garlic, peeled, flattened with the side of a knife blade

2 fresh rosemary sprigs

2 bay leaves

1 tablespoon coriander seeds, coarsely cracked

1 teaspoon dried crushed red pepper

Yield: 4 cups

Place the olives in a medium-size glass or metal bowl. Combine the olive oil, oregano, peppercorns, garlic cloves, rosemary, bay leaves, coriander seeds, and crushed red pepper in a medium, heavy-bottomed saucepan over medium-high heat.

Bring the mixture to a simmer and remove from heat. Remove the bay leaves. Pour the oil mixture over the olives and allow to cool to room temperature. Cover and chill at least 3 days and up to 1 week.

Bring the olives to room temperature. Using a slotted spoon, transfer the olives, herbs, and spices to a serving bowl or a plastic container with a fitting lid. Pour over enough oil from the bowl to coat. Cover the olives and store in the refrigerator for up to 1 week.

Mediterranean Tradition
This recipe makes a great edible gift. Simply package them in pretty containers for their final storage, and they're ready to eat. Chopped, freshly marinated olives are often tossed into blanched vegetables like cauliflower, beans, asparagus, and broccoli, as well as pasta.

Italian Olive Oil and Anchovy Dip/*Bagna cauda*

Literally translated as "hot bath," this dipping sauce for vegetables often appears in the northern Italian region of Piemonte as part of the spring and fall harvest traditions. The fresh, baby vegetables are served with *bagna cauda* the way crudités are served as an appetizer elsewhere. In Piemonte, the dip is served in a traditional terra-cotta dish called a *fujot*. Elsewhere, it may be served in a fondue dish to keep it warm. The vegetables included for serving can be substituted with any seasonal vegetable. Red, yellow, and green pepper strips, snap peas, radishes, and fresh asparagus work well, too.

1 cup (240 ml) finest quality extra-virgin olive oil (unfiltered, if possible)

2 tablespoons (28 g) unsalted butter, room temperature

12 anchovy fillets, drained and rinsed

6 large cloves garlic, chopped

Unrefined sea salt or salt, to taste

Freshly ground black pepper, to taste

1 head radicchio, cut into small wedges

1 pound (455 g) baby carrots

1 pint (230 g) grape tomatoes

1 head broccoli or cauliflower, cut into florets

1 fennel bulb, trimmed and cut into bite-size pieces

1 loaf crusty Italian bread (1 pound, or 455 g), if desired, cut into 2-inch (5 cm) cubes

Yield: 6 servings

Combine the olive oil, butter, anchovies, and garlic in a food processor and blend until smooth.

Transfer the oil mixture to a heavy-bottomed medium saucepan. Cook, uncovered over low heat, 15 minutes, whisking occasionally. (The sauce will separate.) Taste and season with salt and pepper as needed.

Pour the sauce into a warm serving dish or fondue pot. Serve with vegetables and bread, if desired.

Mediterranean Tradition
Olive oil, garlic, and anchovies are a winning combination that taste great and are packed with nutrients. Keep leftover dip in the refrigerator. It tastes great slathered on roasted fish and chicken, and it can even perk up leftovers with its punchy flavor.

Aioli Herb Sauce/*Aioli*

Given the popularity of aioli sauce in upscale restaurants, one would assume that it's a new, cosmopolitan creation. It's actually a traditional Mediterranean condiment that dates back to Phoenician times. Archeologists found it in jars on Phoenician trading ships recently discovered in the Mediterranean Sea. The procedure for making homemade aioli is quick and simple; very similar to making homemade mayonnaise. I add herbs to this version for an even fresher flavor, but you could omit them and add a pinch of saffron or your favorite spice instead.

2 egg yolks

4 cloves garlic, crushed

1 teaspoon white wine vinegar

⅓ cup (80 ml) good-quality, extra-virgin olive oil (unfiltered, if possible)

1 teaspoon fresh tarragon, chopped

1 teaspoon fresh parsley, chopped

1 teaspoon fresh mint, finely chopped

Unrefined sea salt or salt

Freshly ground pepper

Yield: About ½ cup (120 g)

To make the herb aioli by hand, beat the egg yolks, garlic, and vinegar together in a medium-size bowl. Blend in the oil, a few drops at a time, whisking vigorously after each addition, until the aioli is thick and smooth—this may take up to 10 minutes.

Alternately, place the egg yolks, garlic, and vinegar together in a blender and whip until combined. Remove the center spout and carefully pour in the olive oil with the blender running.

Stir in the tarragon, parsley, and mint. Season with salt and pepper to taste.

Mediterranean Tradition

Nowadays, aioli shows up in various guises all around the Mediterranean region. In Spain, it is used as a garnish on potatoes. In Egypt, it is commonly served as an appetizer with pita bread in seafood restaurants. In Greece, the mixture is actually stirred into boiled potatoes and served as a side dish or appetizer called *skordalia*.

Olive Oil-Cured Eggplant/*Melanzane sott'olio*

This easy recipe yields silky, smooth vegetables just begging to be devoured! You will need bags of sugar or flour, or a heavy pot to weigh down the vegetables. Keep in mind that this recipe takes 12 hours inactive time to weigh down the vegetables and another week to fully develop their flavor. This recipe can be made in 1 canning jar (16 ounces, or 475 ml), in 2 jars (8 ounces, or 235 ml, each), or in 4 jars (4 ounces, or 120 ml), each.

3 pounds (1365 g) Japanese eggplant, stemmed and cut into ⅛-inch (3 mm) thick rounds

1 cup (134 g) kosher or sea salt

4 or 5 sprigs fresh oregano, stems trimmed

Handful of fresh, flat-leaf Italian parsley, trimmed

4 cloves garlic, minced

¼ cup (60 ml) red wine vinegar, divided

1 jalapeño pepper

Extra-virgin olive oil

Yield: About 16 ounces (455 g)

In a 9 x 13-inch (23 x 33 cm) plastic or glass container, layer eggplant slices with 2 tablespoons (17 g) of salt scattered over the top of each layer. Cover the container with a lid or a clean kitchen towel. Place the weight on the vegetables. Allow to rest for 12 hours.

Remove the weights, pot, and lid. Add the oregano, parsley, garlic, and 2 tablespoons (30 ml) vinegar. Toss well to coat. Lay the eggplant slices, one on top of the other, in canning the jar until nearly full. Place the pepper on top. With clean fingers, press the eggplant down into the jar. Fill the jar with olive oil and cover. Place in the refrigerator. Eggplant can be eaten the next day, but it takes up to a week for the flavors to fully develop.

Mediterranean Tradition
While the recipe calls for eggplant, any vegetables except for beets and beans (which have very low acidity and yield different results) could be substituted. This type of recipe would be served as an appetizer with other vegetable–based dishes.

Olive Oil and Herb-Marinated Mushrooms/
Funghi sott'olio

This method of pickling mushrooms enables them to be enjoyed the very next day. Keep in mind that any variety of mushrooms or a combination of varieties can be used. Once it is made, this mixture can be preserved in the refrigerator for up to three weeks. White wine or cider vinegar maby be substituted for the balsamic to preserve the natural color of the mushrooms, if desired. Eggplant and zucchini could be substituted for the mushrooms.

1 cup (235 ml) extra-virgin olive oil, divided

4 cloves garlic, sliced

1½ pounds (680 g) chanterelles, shitake, or other mushrooms

½ cup (120 ml) balsamic vinegar

1 teaspoon dried thyme or leaves from 2 fresh thyme sprigs

6 fresh sage leaves, if desired

¼ cup (15 g) chopped fresh parsley

1 bay leaf, crumbled

1 teaspoon pickling salt

½ teaspoon whole black peppercorns

Yield: 2 pint jars

Heat ¼ cup (60 ml) olive oil in a large, wide skillet over medium heat. Add the garlic and allow it to release its aroma. Add the mushrooms and sauté for about 5 to 10 minutes, or until they're tender. Transfer to a bowl.

Pour the vinegar into a small, nonreactive saucepan, Add the herbs, bay leaf, salt, pepper, and remaining ¾ cup (175 ml) of olive oil and bring the mixture just to a boil over high heat.

Pour the mixture over the mushrooms and toss them. Taste and adjust seasoning if necessary.

Divide the mushrooms and their liquid evenly into pint jars. Cap the jars and let them cool to room temperature. Store the mushrooms in the refrigerator for about a week. Bring the jar to room temperature before serving them, stirring, if necessary.

Mediterranean Tradition

Mushrooms are a staple in many of the southern European countries bordering the Mediterranean whose climates are humid enough to grow them. They provide many of the nutritional benefits found in produce, meats, beans, and grains, which is why they are a popular meat substitute. They are low in calories, fat, and are cholesterol free, and they are very low in sodium. They are packed with selenium, potassium, riboflavin, niacin, vitamin D, and more.

Spaghetti with Garlic, Oil, and Chile Pepper/ *Spaghetti al aglio e olio*

Many Italian, first-course, pasta dishes are tossed with fresh vegetables and herbs instead of ladled with a heavy sauce. This spaghetti dish pairs beautifully with heavier, tomato-sauce laden second courses, such as eggplant or chicken parmigiana, or stewed fish, chicken, or meat dishes. This mixture also tastes great drizzled over grilled, steamed, or blanched vegetables.

½ teaspoon kosher or sea salt

1 pound (455 g) spaghetti or gluten-free alternative

¼ cup (60 ml) extra-virgin olive oil, plus extra for drizzling

8 cloves garlic, minced

¼ teaspoon crushed red chili flakes

1 bunch fresh, flat-leaf parsley, finely chopped

⅛ teaspoon freshly ground black pepper

¼ cup (30 g) freshly grated Pecorino cheese

Yield: 8 servings (as a first course)

Bring a large pot of water to a boil over high heat. Add salt. Add the pasta and toss.

Reduce heat to medium-low, and cook, uncovered, until very al dente (see package directions for various pastas), and drain well.

While the pasta is cooking, heat the olive oil in a large, wide skillet over medium heat. Add the garlic and chili flakes, and cook just until they release their aroma, 30 to 60 seconds. Add the pasta and parsley to the skillet, toss to coat. Drizzle with additional olive oil, if desired. Add black pepper to taste and serve immediately with Pecorino cheese.

Mediterranean Tradition

Quick, comforting pasta dishes such as this one are to Italians what pub food is to the Americans and the British. These are the dishes that one eats on occasion to satisfy a craving or to fill one's stomach after a night out with friends. While the carbohydrate-heavy dish isn't the most healthful in this book, it is extremely satisfying, and much more nutritious than fast food. If you don't suffer from gluten sensitivity, seek out pasta made from durum wheat, which offers a higher amount of protein and other nutrients.

Provencal Herb Tapenade/*Tapena*/*Pâté des olives*

The Romans named Provence *Provincia Romana*, or The Roman Province, in Latin when Nice was their capital in the first century CE. The Romans left both vineyards and olive groves as well as the Latin language during their time there. As a result, Provencal cuisine developed strong Italian undertones, as this recipe demonstrates. The word *tapenade* comes from the ancient Provencal word *tapena* which means "to cover." This citrusy olive paste makes the perfect topping for bread, crudités, vegetables, pasta, fish, and chicken.

¾ cup (96 g) pitted black olives (picholine or kalamata work well)

3 teaspoons (26 g) capers, rinsed and drained well

3 cloves garlic, chopped

⅓ cup (80 ml) extra-virgin olive oil, or to taste

1 teaspoon lemon zest

Freshly ground black pepper

Yield: About 1 cup (250 g)

Combine the olives, capers, and garlic in the food processor. Remove the lid of the spout and slowly pour in the olive oil, a little at a time, while pulsing the food processor on and off. The tapenade should have a paste-like consistency, but should not be completely smooth. Stir in the lemon zest and season with freshly ground pepper to taste.

Mediterranean Tradition
Reinventing leftovers into culinary creations is an art form so integral to the region, that it is taken for granted. Leftover roasted chicken or fish and raw vegetables taste great dipped into tapenade. I also like to stir it into blanched green beans that I toss with cucumbers, chickpeas, and cherry tomatoes for a fun and flavorful salad.

Olive, Almond, and Goat Cheese Tapas/
Tapas de aceitunas, almendras y queso de cabra

When eaten 15 minutes before a meal, olives and almonds have been proven to slow digestion and help the body to absorb more nutrients in the upcoming meal. When you add goat cheese into the mix, this appetizer becomes a healthful Mediterranean meal in itself! The almonds and olives can be made a week in advance, and the cheese can be made up to 3 days in advance. Serve with toothpicks or cocktail sticks for spearing the cheese and olives.

For the Almonds:
1 teaspoon Spanish smoked paprika

½ teaspoon unrefined sea salt or salt

½ teaspoon cumin

¼ teaspoon cayenne pepper

¼ cup (60 ml) extra-virgin olive oil

1¾ cups (252 g) blanched almonds

For the Marinated Olives:
1 tablespoon (15 ml) extra-virgin olive oil

1 teaspoon fresh oregano

1 teaspoon fresh parsley

2 cloves garlic, crushed

¼ teaspoon freshly ground black pepper

Pinch crushed red chili flakes

¼ pound (115 g) cured black olives

¼ pound (115 g) cured green olives

For the Marinated Goat Cheese:
5 ounces (140 g) Queso de Murcia, Spanish goat cheese, or any goat cheese

⅓ cup (80 ml) extra-virgin olive oil

Juice and zest of 1 lemon

½ teaspoon black peppercorns

1 clove garlic, minced

Handful of fresh flat-leaf parsley

5 sprigs fresh tarragon

Yield: 6 to 8 servings

To make the almonds: Mix together the paprika, salt, cumin, and cayenne in a small bowl.

Heat the olive oil in a large, wide skillet over medium-high heat. Add the almonds and sauté, stirring constantly, until the almonds begin to turn color and release their aroma, 3 to 5 minutes. Remove from heat, stir in salt mixture and allow to cool. Store in a jar or airtight container for up to 1 week.

To make the marinated olives: Whisk together the olive oil, oregano, parsley, garlic, black pepper, and red chili flakes.

Place the olives in a medium glass bowl or a plastic storage container. Pour the olive oil mixture over the top, mix well to coat, and cover. Store in the refrigerator for up to 1 week.

To make the marinated goat cheese: Shape the cheese into small bite-size balls. Mix together the olive oil, lemon juice and zest, peppercorns, garlic, parsley, and tarragon and pour over the cheese in a medium-size glass bowl or a plastic storage container. Cover and chill for up to 3 days.

Mediterranean Tradition
Hospitality is paramount in all areas of the Mediterranean region, as are impromptu visits. Whenever people are invited into someone else's home as guests, they are immediately given something to eat and drink. Even if guests say that they aren't interested, the items will be brought out and placed in front of them in case they change their mind. Not providing food or drink to guests speaks poorly of the host. To avoid being considered rude, poor, or cheap, people purposely keep special types of appetizers, nibbles, biscuits, and sweets on hand for whomever might drop by. This appetizer trio fits the bill perfectly.

Sweet Olive Oil, Cherry, and Almond Cake/
Torta di ciliegie e mandorle

While this cake is definitely not diet material, I decided to include it in this chapter for two reasons. First, it shows olive oil's versatility, and how delicious it can be in desserts. Second, with the combination of oil, almonds, and fruit, this dessert is actually quite nutritious—and when eaten sparingly can fit into a healthful eating plan. Serve with Vin Santo.

¼ cup (60 ml) extra-virgin olive oil, plus extra

1½ cups (188 g) unbleached all-purpose flour, or all-purpose gluten-free baking mix, or almond flour, plus extra

½ cup (55 g) sliced almonds

2 eggs, separated

⅔ cup (160 ml) freshly squeezed orange juice

2 teaspoons grated orange zest

1 cup (200 g) sugar

2 teaspoons vanilla extract

1 teaspoon almond extract

1 teaspoon orange blossom water

1 teaspoon baking powder

½ teaspoon unrefined sea salt or salt

⅔ cup (64 g) almond flour (or finely ground almonds)

1 cup (155 g) pitted cherries

2 tablespoons (16 g) powdered sugar, to serve

Yield: 9 servings

Preheat the oven to 350°F (180°C). Oil and flour a 9-inch (23 cm) springform pan. Line with a 9-inch (23 cm) round of parchment paper. Brush the parchment paper with olive oil and sprinkle with sliced almonds.

In the bowl of a standing mixer or in a large metal bowl using a hand mixer, beat the egg whites until stiff peaks form.

Combine the orange juice, orange zest, ¼ cup (60 ml) olive oil, egg yolks, sugar, vanilla and almond extracts, and orange blossom water in a medium bowl.

In a large bowl, sift together the ½ cup (188 g) flour, baking powder, salt, and ground almonds. Mix in the orange juice mixture and fold in the cherries.

Pour into the baking pan and smooth out the top with a spatula. Bake until a toothpick inserted into the middle comes out clean and the cake begins to pull away from the sides of the pan, 40 to 45 minutes.

Cool completely. Invert onto a platter, release sides. Remove the parchment paper, sprinkle with powdered sugar, and serve.

Mediterranean Tradition
Seasonal fruit cakes are the cornerstone of every traditional home cook's dessert repertoire in the region. The cherries and almonds could be substituted with figs and walnuts, or blueberries and pecans, depending on the season.

Fish & Seafood: Savoring the Bounty of the Mediterranean Sea

> "*A tavola non si invecchia mai.*" "At the table one never ages."
> —**Italian Proverb**

Sometimes, in the West, fish and seafood get a bad rap. Many people associate them with diet and sacrifice. Their obvious health benefits and low fat content do make them popular with dieters. And for people who have given up meat either for health or spiritual reasons, fish is the go-to substitute. It is rare that one hears of a celebratory meal with fish as a main course.

In countries surrounding the Mediterranean Sea, however, things couldn't be more different. There, serving fish alone is a celebration, and seafood is at the heart of many holidays, from Christmas Eve in Italy to the Eid al Fitr in Egypt. During the Ottoman period (thirteenth to twentieth centuries) in Turkey, there were special chefs called *balikci* who prepared only fish.

The sea and its bounty have always been integral to the livelihood of the region. In addition to providing food, the Mediterranean Sea was an ancient highway that connected continents and enabled trade between countries. To this day, fishing, often even the old-fashioned kind, is an important profession for men in coastal towns, and it is taken very seriously. Fishermen in the region bring their catch to shore early in the morning. Restaurateurs and housewives buy something that was caught within a matter of hours, and cook it the same day. In addition, many fishermen use traditional methods that are more environmentally sound and beneficial to the community.

The reverence that Mediterranean peoples share for bodies of water was evident even in ancient times. Living in harmony with the sea was very important to the cultures of the region. Ancient Egyptians, Greeks, and Romans paid close attention to marine biology, as do their modern descendants—today's Italian news, for example, reports on migratory patterns of fish on a weekly basis.

The ancient Egyptians used to worship a Nile god called Hapi. They believed he was responsible for the biannual flooding of the river that provided natural irrigation—therefore causing a wide variety of produce and grains to flourish. In order to thank Hapi for being so generous, the Egyptians held Nile festivals each July, during which time they forbade anyone to fish or remove anything from the water. Instead, special prayers and incantations were cast into the Nile in a sacred statement of gratitude. When sunset came and the festivities began, people were once again able to take from the Nile. To this day, fish and seafood are beloved foods in Egypt, often incorporated into holidays.

When Greek and Roman powers came to be in Egypt, the Egyptian reverence for the Nile was adapted to the Mediterranean, and many of the ancient deities were associated with the power of the water. With the rise of Christianity, Italians and other coastal dwellers transformed their ancient beliefs into Christian ones. Instead of gods, the locals assigned the Virgin Mary or various saints to their seashores. They would hold special vigils to give thanks to the water, often casting statues, prayers, and flowers onto the water to give thanks for its gifts, just the way the Egyptians had done millennia before. Even today, in many places in the Mediterranean, vigils are held, and communities congregate en masse to pray for fuller nets and to make safe trips.

Nutritional Benefits

The Mediterranean diet recommends eating fish and seafood often, at a minimum of two times per week. High in protein and low in calories, fish is an excellent choice for anyone trying to gain muscle, lose weight, or increase brain function. Fish is full of omega-3 fatty acids, which the body requires to function, yet cannot produce on its own. They are known to lower triglycerides and blood pressure, and reduce blood clotting and risk of stroke and heart failure.

Consuming fish as little as once a week promotes body wellness and positive health benefits. But a 2011 study found that a single extra serving of fish per week can reduce heart disease risk by 50 percent. According to Hypertension: Journal of the American Heart Association, women who didn't eat fish regularly had 50 percent more heart problems, three times greater risk for disease, and higher blood fat levels than those who did.

In addition to omega-3s, seafood has essential nutrients such as zinc (immune-system support), potassium (heart health), selenium (anti-cancer protection), and iodine (for thyroid function), along with vitamins A (vision, organ function, immune support) and D (bone strength, nutrient absorption, disease prevention). Additional benefits of omega-3 and fish consumption have been shown to:

- potentially lower the risk of Alzheimer's disease, dementia, and decreased cognitive function
- subdue the symptoms of ADHD (poor concentration, reading skills, and negative behavior)
- relieve and prevent asthma symptoms
- keep skin nourished and hair lustrous
- help reverse UV damage from sun exposure
- enhance mood, including depression, postpartum depression, and Seasonal Affective Disorder
- protect the vision of those suffering from Age-Related Macular Degeneration
- prevent inflammation and improve rheumatoid arthritis

With all of these healthful reasons to consume more fish, many still avoid it altogether for fear of mercury levels and unclean water. When purchasing fish, one has to take mercury levels, health benefits, and the water sources into account in order to make an informed decision. With no single guide currently available to analyze all three factors, the Environmental Defense Fund does produce a Seafood Selector, and Monterey Bay Aquarium created a Seafood Watch program that addresses mercury levels and water cleanliness. I am an advocate of the freshest local seafood possible, or imports from safe sources. I strongly encourage shoppers to educate themselves as much as possible to make the best choices and reap the most health rewards.

A serving size of fish is 3.5 ounces (100 g). I've developed quick-cooking recipes with maximum flavor and health benefits that win over even the toughest critics. With these simple, flavorful, and healthful recipes, seafood will become an easy go-to meal for a busy weeknight. For safety reasons, cook seafood to an internal temperature of 145°F (63°C) for 15 seconds, or until flaky, opaque, and no longer translucent.

Moroccan-Style Grilled Tuna/*Samak bil Chermoula*

When we think of Moroccan cuisine, lamb, couscous, and tajines usually come to mind. Bordering both the Mediterranean Sea and Atlantic Ocean, however, Morocco offers a wonderful array of flavors from the sea. This recipe features *chermoula* sauce, a Moroccan classic that tastes great on both chicken and fish. If you prefer to make this dish in the oven, instead of grilling it, simply place the fish in a greased baking dish, top with chermoula, cover with aluminum foil, and bake in a 425°F (220°C) oven for 20 to 25 minutes, or until cooked through.

2 tablespoons (2 g) finely chopped cilantro

2 tablespoons (8 g) finely chopped parsley

6 cloves garlic, minced

½ teaspoon unrefined sea salt or salt

½ teaspoon paprika

1 lemon, juiced and zested

3 tablespoons (45 ml) extra-virgin olive oil

4 tuna steaks (4 ounces, or 115 g each)

Yield: 4 servings

In a medium bowl, mix the cilantro, parsley, garlic, salt, paprika, and lemon juice and zest together. Whisk in the olive oil.

Place the fish in a glass baking dish and pour half of the chermoula sauce over the top. Cover with plastic wrap and allow to marinate for 1 hour.

Preheat grill to medium-high heat.

Grill the fish, turning once, until firm, 6 to 8 minutes. Transfer to a platter, spread with the remaining chermoula sauce, and let stand for 5 minutes to absorb the flavors.

Mediterranean Tradition

Marinating seafood, meat, and chicken before grilling it not only flavors it, it also reduces the harmful cancer-causing substances that can be caused by cooking over an open flame.

Greek-Style Roasted Fish and Vegetables/*Psari Plaki*

Psari Plaki means "baked fish" in Greek. This recipe is a traditional Greek-style fish that is baked with a variety of savory ingredients—making it a perfect meal in one. Popular throughout Greece nowadays, this dish is made from a wide variety of fish including salted cod, sea bass, mullet, halibut, and red snapper. For convenience, fish fillets can be substituted, and freshwater fish from lakes, such as trout, is also often used.

¼ cup (60 ml) extra olive oil, plus 1 teaspoon, divided

1 bunch of fresh parsley, chopped

4 medium Yukon gold potatoes (2 pounds, or 910 g), cut into wedges

2 Cubanelle peppers, sliced into rings

2 medium tomatoes, diced

3 cloves garlic, roughly chopped, plus 2 additional cloves, chopped, if using whole fish

¼ cup (16 g) fresh oregano, finely chopped, or 1 tablespoon (3 g) dried

1 whole fish such as cod or red snapper (2½ pounds, or 1.1 kg), scaled and gutted

or

6 cod, red snapper, sea bass, or halibut fillets (⅓ pound, or 152 g, each)

1 medium tomato, halved and cut into slices

2 tablespoons (16 g) unbleached, all-purpose flour

1 teaspoon sweet paprika

Unrefined sea salt or salt

Freshly ground pepper

Yield: 6 servings

Preheat the oven to 350°F (180°C). Grease the bottom of a large baking dish with 1 teaspoon olive oil. Place a handful of freshly chopped parsley, potatoes, pepper slices, diced tomatoes, 3 cloves garlic, and 1 tablespoon (4 g) oregano on the bottom of the pan, layering each one on top of the other.

If using a whole fish: Season the fish (inside and out) with salt and pepper and fill the cavity with remaining garlic, parsley, and oregano. Place the fish on the bed of herbs and vegetables, and arrange the slices of tomatoes around the fish.

If using fillets: Season with salt and pepper and lay on top of vegetable mixture. Arrange the slices of tomatoes around the fish.

Add the remaining ¼ cup (60 ml) of olive oil, flour, and paprika into a small bowl or measuring cup and whisk vigorously to incorporate. Pour the mixture over the fish. Pour ½ cup (120 ml) of water over all the herbs and vegetables on the sides of the pan.

Season with salt and ground pepper, and bake 40 to 45 minutes for whole fish or 20 to 25 minutes for fillets, or until the fish is opaque and flakes easily when pierced with a fork. Carefully remove the fish from the baking dish and serve each plate with a fillet of the fish on top of a bed of vegetables. Spoon the sauce from the baking dish over the top and sides to finish.

Mediterranean Tradition
Greek cooks will often change and substitute ingredients depending on availability and personal tastes. A common addition, which I have left out of this version, is raisins, which give a sweet and sour flavor to the fish. Serve this dish with a small piece of feta cheese, olives, crusty bread, and a tossed salad dressed with extra-virgin olive oil and lemon juice.

Italian Halibut with Grapes and Olive Oil/
Pesce al forno con l'uva

Creative chefs in Italian coastal regions sometimes replace grapes for the tomatoes in a dish called *pesce in acqua pazza* or "fish in crazy water." It's called crazy water because crushed red chilies give the cooking water a kick. Typically, freshly caught sea bream is used, although I have substituted halibut for its easy access and high omega-3 content in this recipe. It's said that this dish can transport someone from a rainy day in London to the sunny Italian Riviera.

¼ cup (60 ml) extra-virgin olive oil

4 boneless halibut fillets, 4 ounces (115 g) each

4 cloves garlic, roughly chopped

1 small red chile pepper, finely chopped

2 cups (300 g) seedless green grapes

A handful of fresh basil leaves, roughly torn

½ teaspoon unrefined sea salt or salt

Freshly ground black pepper

Yield: 4 servings

Heat the olive oil in a large, heavy-bottomed skillet over medium-high heat. Add the halibut, followed by the garlic, chile pepper, grapes, basil, and the salt and pepper. Pour in 1¾ cups (410 ml) of water, turn the heat down to medium-low, cover, and cook the fish until opaque, or for 7 minutes on each side.

Remove the fish from the pan and place on a large serving dish. Raise the heat, cook the sauce for 30 seconds to concentrate the flavors slightly. Taste and adjust salt and pepper. Pour sauce over the fish.

Mediterranean Tradition
Phytonutrients in grapes are believed to contribute to longevity. Try incorporating them into recipes for a surprising fresh, sweet and sour flavor.

Sicilian Swordfish Bundles/*Involtini di pesce spada*

Swordfish is one of the most traditional fish in the southern Italian diet. Although it can be eaten at any time of year, it is often a part of the Feast of the Seven Fishes custom celebrated on Christmas Eve (see Mediterranean Tradition).

4 tablespoons (60 ml) extra-virgin olive oil, divided

2 cloves garlic, minced

1 cup (226 g) chopped boxed tomatoes, such as Pomi brand

1 cup (226 g) strained boxed tomatoes, such as Pomi brand

4 tablespoons (36 g) toasted pine nuts, divided

2 tablespoons (5 g) freshly chopped basil

½ teaspoon unrefined sea salt or salt, divided

⅛ teaspoon freshly ground black pepper

Dash of crushed dried red chili flakes

2 boneless swordfish fillets (¾ pound, or 340 g), placed in freezer for 30 minutes for easier slicing

2 tablespoons (6 g) Fresh Bread Crumbs (see page 182)

2 tablespoons (15 g) grated Pecorino Romano

2 tablespoons (18 g) raisins, soaked in warm water for 20 minutes and drained

1 tablespoon (10 g) finely chopped onion

2 tablespoons (8 g) chopped fresh, flat-leaf Italian parsley, divided

¼ cup (22 g) finely chopped fennel

2 anchovy fillets, chopped

Yield: 4 servings

Heat 2 tablespoons (30 ml) of olive oil in a large skillet over medium heat. Add the garlic and cook until it releases its aroma, 30 to 60 seconds—do not let garlic turn brown.

Stir in the chopped and strained tomatoes, 2 tablespoons (18 g) pine nuts, basil, ¼ teaspoon salt, pepper, and chili flakes, stir, and cover. Reduce heat to low and simmer for 5 minutes.

With a filleting knife, carefully and neatly slice the swordfish fillets crosswise once into about ⅛-inch (3 mm) thick slices. Cut each piece in half to make 4 pieces.

Combine the remaining 2 tablespoons (30 ml) of olive oil, bread crumbs, Pecorino, raisins, remaining pine nuts, remaining salt, onion, parsley, fennel, and anchovies in a small bowl, and mix well to combine.

Place the fish pieces on a work surface covered with waxed paper or on a large plastic cutting board, and spread 1 tablespoon (12 g) of the bread crumb mixture on each piece of fish. Press down firmly with your hands, so that the filling sticks.

Carefully tuck in the sides of fish. The sides must be firmly tucked in so that the filling doesn't escape. Starting at the wide end, roll up the fish, completely encasing the filling. Use toothpicks or skewers to secure the rolls.

Slowly remove lid from tomato sauce and add the rolls into simmering sauce. Cover and cook for 15 to 20 minutes, turning once, or until fish is cooked through.

Transfer the fish to a serving platter, remove skewers, and top with the remaining sauce.

Mediterranean Tradition

While not everyone in Italy adheres to the Feast of the Seven Fishes menu on Christmas Eve, many do. The Feast consists of a dinner with seven courses, all created from fish and seafood. The number of courses or type of fish served at the meal is open to interpretation. Some maintain that the number seven stands for the seven sacraments, and others say it refers to the number of days it took God to create the universe. Other variations on the Feast call for nine types of fish to be served, signifying the Holy Trinity times three, and still others say the correct number is thirteen, for the twelve apostles and Jesus.

Trout Cooked in Parchment/*Trota al cartoccio*

Moist and flavorful, this easy-to-clean cooking method is popular all over Italy. Trout is one of the fish with some of the highest amounts of omega-3s.

4 (4 ounces, or 115 g, each) trout fillets

3 cloves garlic, finely chopped

8 fresh sage leaves, finely chopped

½ cup (30 g) finely chopped fresh parsley

Zest and juice of 1 lemon

⅓ cup (80 ml) extra-virgin olive oil

1 teaspoon unrefined sea salt or salt

Freshly ground pepper

Lemon wedges

Yield: 4 servings

Preheat the oven to 425°F (220°C). Combine the garlic, sage, parsley, lemon zest and juice, olive oil, salt, and pepper in a small bowl. Cut four pieces of parchment paper—each more than double the size of the trout.

Place 1 trout on top of each piece of parchment and equally distribute ¼ of garlic herb mixture on each fish. Brush any remaining garlic herb mixture over the fish and fold the parchment over the fish. Fold and crimp the edges to seal tightly and place in a baking dish.

Bake about 10 minutes, until fish is cooked through. Remove from the oven, and serve with lemon wedges, allowing guests to open their own individual packages at the table.

Mediterranean Tradition
Thinly sliced vegetables such as fennel, eggplant, tomatoes, and zucchini could be baked alongside the fish in the parchment.

Citrus-Marinated Salmon with Fennel Cream/
Salmone agli agrumi con crema di finocchio

Orange and salmon are a match made in heaven. The sweet citrus flavors combine with the rich, oily textures in the salmon for a healthful dish that seems too decadent to be good for you. Fennel and yogurt are two popular Mediterranean ingredients that are as virtuous as they are delicious.

2 tablespoons (30 ml) extra-virgin olive oil

¼ cup (60 ml) orange juice

½ teaspoon unrefined sea salt or salt

Freshly ground pepper

4 salmon fillets (4 ounces, or 115 g, each), skin-on

1 fennel bulb, thinly sliced (reserve fronds)

½ sweet onion, thinly sliced

1 cup (230 g) plain Greek yogurt

2 oranges, 1 zested, 1 thinly sliced

Yield: 4 servings

In a small bowl, whisk the olive oil, orange juice, salt, and pepper together until emulsified.

Place the salmon fillets in a glass baking dish and pour marinade over the top. Allow to marinate for 1 hour.

Preheat the oven to 400°F (200°C).

Scatter fennel and onion around the sides of the salmon, and cover the baking dish with aluminum foil. Bake until the fish flakes easily with a fork and is opaque in color, 20 to 25 minutes.

While the fish is baking, combine the Greek yogurt with 2 tablespoons (6 g) fennel fronds, finely chopped, and orange zest.

Remove the fish from oven and place on a serving plate. Dollop each with about ¼ of yogurt mixture and garnish with orange slices.

Mediterranean Tradition
Fennel, known to be a digestive aid, is often eaten raw in salads, braised, or roasted as in recipes such as this one. Its seeds are also used as a spice and boiled to make soothing after-dinner teas.

Mussels in Tomato-Saffron Broth/*Moules Provencales*

If you've never made mussels before, you'll be surprised at how easy it is. Buy the freshest mussels possible, preferably the day you're using them. If your local purveyor only sells muscles in a mesh bag, buy more than you need, as the bags make it seem as if all the mussels crammed into it are closed (living), but this isn't always the case. Scrub mussels with a clean kitchen brush and rinse under cold water. Use only mussels that are closed and have no cracks. (If a mussel is only slightly open, tap it on the kitchen counter; if it closes up within a minute or two, it is safe to use.)

¼ cup (60 ml) extra-virgin olive oil

2 teaspoons fresh thyme

2 teaspoons fresh oregano

1 teaspoon fennel seeds, crushed in a mortar to release aroma

¼ teaspoon saffron

2 cloves garlic, minced

½ teaspoon fresh orange zest

½ pound (225 g) tomatoes, peeled and diced

2 cups (475 ml) Seafood Stock (see page 183)

½ teaspoon unrefined sea salt or salt, to taste

Freshly ground pepper

1 pound (455 g) fresh mussels, scrubbed and beards removed

¼ cup (15 g) fresh parsley, finely chopped, for garnish

Yield: 4 servings

Heat the olive oil in a large stockpot over medium heat. Add the thyme, oregano, fennel, saffron, garlic, and orange zest, and cook, uncovered, until the garlic begins to release its aroma, 1 to 2 minutes.

Stir in the tomatoes, stock, salt, and pepper, and bring to a boil over high heat.

Stir, add in the mussels, cover, and cook for 7 to 10 minutes, until the mussels are open completely. Resist the urge to open the cover and check the mussels often. Each time you release steam it adds on to the cooking time and could yield tough mussels. I usually check the first time by carefully removing the lid with the steam releasing away from me. If mussels aren't open, I quickly recover them, and allow them to cook for a few more minutes.

When mussels are ready, they are completely open. If you have some open mussels and other closed ones, remove the cooked ones with a ladle and allow the rest to continue to cook. If any still refuse to open after 10 minutes, discard them.

Taste the broth, and adjust salt and pepper if necessary. Pour into individual cups or bowls, and add mussels. Sprinkle the tops with fresh parsley. I like to serve it with toasted bread crostini slathered with Aioli Herb Sauce (page 95).

Mediterranean Tradition
The ingredients in this recipe are based on my favorite version of the classic southern French seafood stew, bouillabaisse. To make your own seafood stew, simply double the ingredients for the broth used above. In addition to the pound (455 g) of mussels, add ½ pound (225 g) shelled shrimp, ½ pound (225 g) firm white fish, such as cod or halibut, cut into 1-inch (2.5 cm) cubes into the pot at the same time that you add the mussels. Everything should be done at the same time, and you'll have a Mediterranean seafood feast in minutes.

Sizzling Rosemary Shrimp over Polenta/
Gamberi al rosmarino con polenta

Think of this recipe as the Mediterranean cousin of shrimp and grits. The savory, flash-sautéed shrimp taste great on their own as a tapa along with the Olive, Almond, and Goat Cheese Tapas (page 101), or tossed into spaghetti or linguine with olive oil and lemon zest. Serving them over polenta, a traditional staple in Italy since the sixteenth century, rounds out the meal.

¼ cup (60 ml) extra-virgin olive oil

2 cloves garlic, minced

1½ pounds (680 g) prawns or jumbo shrimp, peeled and deveined

2 teaspoons freshly chopped rosemary

Dash of crushed red chili flakes

½ teaspoon kosher salt

¼ teaspoon freshly ground black pepper

3 cups cooked polenta (see page 182)

Yield: 6 Servings

Heat the olive oil in a large skillet over medium-high heat. Add the garlic and stir. Add the prawns or shrimp, rosemary, chili flakes, salt, and pepper.

Cook, uncovered, for about 2 minutes per side, or until prawns or shrimp turn pink. Spoon the polenta onto a serving platter evenly, and flatten with the back of a spoon. Place prawns or shrimp on the top of the plate and serve immediately.

Mediterranean Tradition
Known for a wide variety of health benefits, fresh and dried rosemary along with rosemary oil, tonics, and tea are used daily in the Mediterranean. It is believed that its aroma boosts brain power. It also possesses antiviral properties and is known to relieve pain and ease menstrual disorders, kidney stones, and digestion, as well as increase the appetite and help with gall bladder, liver, and heart problems. Rosemary oil is massaged into the scalp for stronger, darker hair and to alleviate dandruff and skin problems.

Greek Island-Style Stuffed Calamari with Rice and Herbs/*Yemisto Kalamari me Voutiro*

Baby squid are surprisingly simple to prepare. If you've only eaten fried calamari, you'll love this light, healthful version with its flavors are straight from the Aegean Islands. The tender texture of the calamari in this unique dish lends itself to a straightforward cooking style. You may also cook full-size squid this way, but you will need to increase the filling quantities and cooking time.

2 tablespoons (30 ml) extra-virgin olive oil, divided

1 small yellow onion, finely chopped

1 pound (455 g) fresh spinach

¼ cup (50 g) short-grain rice

2 tablespoons (8 g) freshly chopped parsley

2 tablespoons (15 g) freshly chopped dill

1 teaspoon unrefined sea salt or salt

Freshly ground pepper

Dash of crushed red chili flakes

1 pound (455 g) baby squid, tentacles removed, and cleaned

2 cups (475 ml) Vegetable or Seafood Stock (see page 183)

Yield: 4 servings

Heat 1 tablespoon (15 ml) of olive oil in a large, wide skillet over medium heat. Add the onion and sauté until golden, about 5 minutes.

Add the spinach, rice, parsley, dill, salt, pepper, and red chili flakes and cook for 1 minute. Take the mixture off the heat and allow to cool slightly.

Stuff the calamari three-quarters of the way full with stuffing. Secure the top with a toothpick, leaving a little bit of room between the toothpick and the top of the stuffing for the rice to expand while cooking.

Heat the remaining olive oil in a large frying pan over medium heat. Brown the calamari on all sides.

Add the stock, cover, and simmer on low until cooked through, 15 to 20 minutes, or until the rice is tender to the bite and the calamari are cooked through. Serve warm.

Mediterranean Tradition

Squid is one of the varieties of seafood that is high in cholesterol, yet if cholesterol is not a concern, it is a great choice because of its high vitamin and mineral content. Squid is very high in copper, a trace mineral that helps the body with nutrient absorption. A great source of complete protein, squid is good for burning fat and building muscle. The high B_2 content makes it an effective pain reliever that helps relieve migraine symptoms.

Citrus-Marinated Scallops/
Capesante marinate al limone

This delicious and impressive dish can be cooked in minutes and served as an appetizer or main course. These scallops also taste great when tossed into a salad or pasta, rice, and other grain-based dishes. In the United States, scallops are sometimes soaked in the preservative trisodium phosphate (TSP), which makes them weigh more, and consequently cost more. TSP also makes scallops exude moisture as they cook, thereby causing them to steam rather than sear properly. Look for scallops labeled dry, that is, not soaked in TSP.

Juice and zest of 2 lemons

¼ cup (60 ml) extra-virgin olive oil

Unrefined sea salt or salt, to taste

Freshly ground black pepper, to taste

1 clove garlic, minced

1½ pounds (680 g) dry scallops, side muscle removed

Yield: 4 servings

In a large shallow bowl or baking dish, combine the lemon juice and zest, olive oil, salt, pepper, and garlic. Mix well to combine. Add the scallops to the marinade; cover and refrigerate 1 hour.

Heat a large skillet over medium-high heat. Drain the scallops and place them in skillet. Cook 4 to 5 minutes per side, until cooked through.

Mediterranean Tradition

All throughout the region, scallops are increasingly being enjoyed raw in beautiful *carpaccios*. To make a carpaccio, simply place the scallops on a baking sheet lined with waxed paper. Cover with plastic wrap and place in the freezer for at least 1 hour. When the scallops are almost hard, remove them from the freezer and with a sharp filleting knife, carefully cut the scallops widthwise into paper-thin slices. Place them on a platter. Drizzle with a vinaigrette and serve with greens. Note that consuming raw or undercooked seafood and shellfish may increase your risk of food-borne illness.

Dairy & Poultry: Farm-Fresh Flavors

"*Non si fanno frittate senza rompere le uova.*" "You can't make an omelet without breaking eggs." **You have to take action, if you want to bring about change.**

Chicken and eggs don't usually conjure up images of luxury in today's world. Readily available and packed with protein, these two culinary staples are the backbone of kitchens everywhere. In the Mediterranean region, they are greatly appreciated and prepared in scores of ways. Believe it or not, up until the last few centuries, both chicken and eggs were quite expensive and reserved for special occasions. During the late sixteenth century, for example, King Henry IV of France told the citizens of his country that his goal was to enable each French family to afford a single chicken for their Sunday supper. "A chicken in every pot" became a political slogan in France, and roasted chicken has been considered a classic Sunday lunch dish.

Further east in the Mediterranean, however, Ottoman–controlled Egypt was extremely wealthy thanks to the spice trade. In thirteenth and fourteenth century Egypt, a single banquet consisted of thousands of animals and tons of sugar for desserts and sorbets. Free hospitals treated needy patients and did not release them until they could eat an entire roasted chicken by themselves, in one sitting.

Many egg-based dishes traveled throughout the region with the migrating Sephardic Jewish diaspora. Since kosher laws weren't adhered to in many countries in the Mediterranean, members of the Jewish community often relied on eggs for their main source of protein, omitting the need to purchase nonkosher meat. These recipes, while inexpensive, are often so delicious that they are preferred to nonvegetarian alternatives. Regardless of the history and lore surrounding these ingredients, dairy, eggs, and poultry are blank culinary canvases that, with passionate Mediterranean flair, can be transformed into inexpensive and healthful edible masterpieces.

DAIRY

A trip to any Mediterranean country is a dairy lover's dream. With most nations offering hundreds of local varieties, there's something for everyone's palate.

Cheese has become a culinary ambassador of sorts, for many countries. It's hard to think of the French kitchen without images of tangy goat cheese and golden brie coming to mind. Fresh mozzarella, Pecorino, and Parmigiano are associated with Italian food. The feta of Greece, Halloumi of Crete, and Kasseri of Turkey continue to grow in popularity around the globe.

To our knowledge, there are at least 900 varieties of artisanal cheeses in the world. Many cheeses have been made in the same artisanal fashion for centuries, ensuring authenticity, flavor, and environmentally sound practices. Great care goes into making artisan cheese. Ancient farming practices that emphasize the wellbeing of the animals include high-quality feed, grazing in cooler pastures in the hot summer months, and hand milking. In the European portion of the Mediterranean region, many of these types of cheese are given a government seal of approval, promoted as culinary treasures, and controlled for quality. In other countries, such as Lebanon and Israel, there are groups of proud farmers, chefs, and their supporters who are working diligently to continue the traditions of the past.

Goat, sheep, cow, buffalo, and in some areas of the Middle East, camel's milk are made into a wide variety of cheeses, which fall into three categories:

- fresh and soft (water content between 45 percent and 70 percent with a lower sodium content)
- semi-hard (water content between 40 percent and 45 percent)
- hard and aged (water content below 40 percent and higher sodium content)

The manner in which cheese is consumed varies from place to place. In France and Italy, cheese courses are served after a meal. In Spain and Greece, cheese features prominently in the small plate, tapas, or meze dining culture. In North Africa and the Middle East, cheese is predominately eaten at breakfast or in sandwiches for a snack or light dinner. The North African and Middle Eastern countries also tend to not add cheese to recipes, but to eat it on its own, in its original form.

Similarly, while many types of yogurt are available and eaten throughout the region, the various Mediterranean cultures have their own uses for yogurt. It was originally made by Bedouins who poured camel, sheep, goat, or ewe's milk into canvas hides tied between two palm trees. The hides would be shaken back and forth until the milk thickened into yogurt. Yogurt cheese and dried yogurt balls were then made and preserved to last without refrigeration. This was a traditional staple of the people of the Middle East whose daily diet was rounded out with dates and bread.

Fresh yogurt is used as a condiment, served for breakfast, used as the base of cold soups and sauces, and a popular snack. Smooth, creamy, and known for cultivating friendly intestinal bacteria, yogurt is an ingredient that seems to prove more beneficial each day.

Nutritional Benefits

Dairy often gets excluded from many western healthy eating plans because people either consume too much milk, which leads to gastric distress, or high-fat butter and processed cheeses, which are also high in cholesterol. Daily consumption of dairy in the Mediterranean region, in contrast, consists of fresh cheeses such as ricotta and feta, which are high in nutrients and lower in fat and cholesterol. To wit, a Spanish study concluded that those eating two to three servings, or more, of low-fat dairy had a 50 percent reduced risk of developing high blood pressure, while a University of Tennessee, Knoxville, study found that the calcium in yogurt, eaten in addition to cutting overall calories, made it easier for participants to drop pounds.

Milk and its products contain a healthful dose of animal protein (about 9 grams per 6-ounce (170 g) serving), plus other nutrients such as calcium, vitamin B_2, B_{12}, potassium, and magnesium. Calcium has been shown to have beneficial effects on bone mass in people of all ages, but check nutritional labels to choose brands of milk and yogurt that contain at least 20 percent of the daily recommended value of both calcium and vitamin D. (Because vitamin D boosts calcium absorption, but isn't naturally present in dairy, most western companies add it.) Nutritional values of traditional yogurt in the Mediterranean region also vary since it can be made from goat, sheep, or cow's milk, or a combination.

Yogurt with live active cultures (probiotics) helps to maintain the natural balance of organisms, known as microflora, in the intestines. According to researchers at Tufts University, yogurt with active cultures is believed to boost the immune system, change the microflora of the gut, and affect the amount of time it takes for food to travel through the bowel. Digestive concerns such as lactose intolerance, constipation, diarrhea, colon cancer, *H. pylori* infections, and inflammatory bowel disease have been shown to improve with probiotic consumption.

Yogurt, especially the Greek variety and type that is locally produced in many Mediterranean countries, is packed with protein and vitamin B_{12}, which is mostly found in animal products, making it a great choice for

vegetarians and for athletes looking for a post-workout snack. The protein helps muscle recovery and water absorption, which can improve hydration. One 8-ounce (225 g) serving contains approximately 60 percent of the recommended daily B_{12} intake for adult women along with good amounts of phosphorus, potassium, riboflavin, iodine, zinc, and vitamin B_5.

Cheese is also a great source of hunger-curbing protein and calcium. It is believed to slow down the absorption rate of carbohydrates eaten at the same meal, balance blood sugar levels, and improve mood. It also contains the same calcium benefits as milk and yogurt. The zinc content in cheese is believed to protect skin, hair, and nails, as well as help tissue growth and repair.

Cypriot Halloumi, Watermelon, and Basil Kabobs/ *Haloumi Souvlaki me Karpouzi ke Vasiliko*

Halloumi is a soft, salty cheese with herbal undertones that has been crafted on the island of Cyprus since antiquity. Artisan Halloumi cheese is still made of sheep and goat's milk the way it was millennia ago. On the island of Cyprus, watermelon is paired with feta cheese for a sweet and salty combination that can't be beat. It's the perfect after dinner treat to enjoy with friends on a balmy evening.

2 cups (300 g) watermelon cubes (1 inch, or 2.5 cm)

1 pound (455 g) Halloumi cheese, cut into 1-inch (2.5 cm) cubes

1 bunch fresh basil

¼ cup (60 ml) good-quality extra-virgin olive oil

Short wooden skewers, for serving

Yield: 8 servings

Thread a piece of watermelon onto a skewer. Follow with a piece of halloumi and a basil leaf. Continue until all of the watermelon and Halloumi have been used up.
   Drizzle with olive oil.

Mediterranean Tradition
The base of the Mediterranean Diet Pyramid emphasizes eating meals with others, and Cyprus is the perfect place to do it! Local *tavernas* offer dozens (often as many as fifty-four) of *mezedes,* or small plates, to groups of friends who spend hours at the table slowly savoring the delicious treats.

Middle Eastern Cottage Cheese, Vegetable, and Olive Salad/*Salata gebna arayish*

I spent a great deal of time in Egypt both consulting for restaurants, visiting loved ones, and as the Chairperson of the Baltimore-Luxor-Alexandria Sister City organization, which promoted cross-cultural relations between the United States and Egypt. Two of my proudest moments were obtaining a grant to give clean water to a rural village outside of Luxor, and creating the menu for a dinner that was attended by the Governor of Luxor and the Mayor of Baltimore. Over the years, Egypt became a third home to me, and when I am not there, I often crave its cuisine.

3 cups (675 g) small curd cottage cheese

1 tomato, chopped

1 baby (Persian) cucumber, or ⅓ English cucumber, diced

¼ cup (32 g) kalamata olives, pitted and chopped

Unrefined sea salt or salt, to taste

Freshly ground black pepper, to taste

¼ cup (60 ml) extra-virgin olive oil (unfiltered if possible)

¼ cup (15 g) chopped fresh parsley

6 pieces Whole-Wheat Pita Bread, quartered (see page 19)

or

Raw vegetables for serving

Yield: 6 servings

Combine the cottage cheese, tomato, cucumber, and olives in a medium bowl. Toss gently to combine. Taste, and season with salt and pepper, if needed. Place the cottage cheese on a dinner plate, and using a spatula, smooth out the top. Drizzle olive oil on the top and garnish with parsley. Serve with pita wedges or crudités.

Mediterranean Tradition

This healthy salad is eaten for breakfast in Egypt and other places in the eastern Mediterranean. Savory breakfasts are a way that many North African and Eastern European communities start their day. When you're in the mood for a Mediterranean–inspired brunch or vegetarian meal, serve with Herb-Marinated Olives (page 93), Israeli *Shakshouka*-Style Eggs (page 153), Whole-Wheat Pita Bread (page 19), and Cypriot Greengrocer's Salad (page 138) for a cornucopia of healthful flavors.

Turkish Yogurt, Garlic, and Dill Sauce/*Cacik*

Yogurt is one of the traditional pleasures of kitchens around the Mediterranean. It's usually enjoyed for breakfast, or a light snack, with fresh figs and luscious mountain honey. For best results, drain the yogurt overnight. After draining the yogurt, enjoy the excess liquid, or whey, as a refreshing drink. It is full of healthful probiotic nutrients, and good bacteria known to aid digestion.

3 cups (690 g) plain organic full-fat yogurt

2 English cucumbers, peeled and diced

Unrefined sea salt or salt

¼ cup (16 g) fresh dill, chopped

1 clove garlic, minced

1 small yellow onion, grated and drained

Yield: 8 servings

Place the yogurt in a medium colander over a bowl to drain overnight in the refrigerator.

Place the cucumbers in a colander and sprinkle with ¼ teaspoon salt. Let stand for 20 minutes. Rinse off the salt and add cucumbers to yogurt. Stir in the dill. Add the garlic and onion, and season with salt to taste. Serve immediately to prevent salad from becoming runny. If storing, place in an airtight container in the refrigerator and drain off excess liquid before serving.

Mediterranean Tradition
This type of sauce is considered a salad in the region. It can be eaten with pita at breakfast time, or as a garnish for kabobs or grilled meats.

Herb-Marinated Mozzarella/*Mozzarella marinata*

This Italian classic makes a tasty and beautiful appetizer or edible gift. Feel free to alter the recipe, using the herbs you have on hand. Garlic, capers, chopped olives, and hot peppers are all popular additions. You can also use larger pieces of mozzarella, instead of bocconcini, and slice them into ¼-inch (6 mm) slices.

¼ cup (60 ml) good-quality, extra-virgin olive oil

1 teaspoon finely chopped fresh flat-leaf parsley

1 teaspoon finely chopped fresh basil

1 teaspoon finely chopped fresh oregano

¼ teaspoon crushed red pepper flakes

¼ teaspoon unrefined sea salt or salt

Pinch freshly ground black pepper

1 pound (455 g) fresh bocconcini mozzarella balls, preferably from buffalo milk

Olives and crackers or bread to serve

Yield: 6 servings

In a small bowl, combine the oil, herbs, red pepper flakes, salt, and pepper. Place the mozzarella balls in a shallow bowl. Drizzle the oil and herb mixture over mozzarella. Let stand for an hour. Serve with olives, crackers, and bread.

Mediterranean Tradition
Buffalos were introduced to the Campania region of Italy via Egypt in antiquity. Their rich, sweet milk has been used to produce deeply flavored butter and cheese ever since. These mozzarella balls are a great stir-in to pastas and salads when the temperature is too high to spend a long time in the kitchen. If buffalo-milk mozzarella is not available in your area, look for the freshest variety possible.

Homemade Yogurt Cheese/*Labneh*

It's surprisingly simple to make Lebanon's namesake yogurt cheese. Since there are only a few ingredients in this recipe, quality ingredients are paramount. Choose the best quality yogurt you can find, preferably one made of sheep and goat's milk cheese from a Mediterranean import store. I also suggest drizzling with unfiltered olive oil, if possible. Some people add finely diced celery, radishes, carrots, or tomatoes to their labneh, but I'm a purist and prefer it plain. Be sure to save the strained liquid—it contains all of the healthful probiotics from the yogurt and makes a great addition to smoothies.

4 cups (920 g) full-fat plain yogurt

1 teaspoon unrefined sea salt or salt

Good-quality, extra-virgin olive oil, unfiltered, if possible

Za'atar (see page 185)

6 to 8 black olives

Whole-Wheat Pita Bread (page 19) or other bread, for serving

Yield: about 2 cups

Line a nonreactive strainer with a few layers of cheesecloth and set it over a deep bowl, one deep enough so that the bottom of the strainer is a 2 to 3 inches (5 to 7.5 cm) above the bottom of the bowl where the strained liquid (whey) will collect.

Stir a teaspoon of salt into the yogurt. Using a spatula, scrape the yogurt into the lined strainer. Fold the ends of the cheesecloth over the yogurt and refrigerate overnight, or for a minimum of 12 hours.

Remove the thickened strained cheese (labneh) from the cloth. Transfer the mixture to a shallow serving dish and smooth out the top in a circular fashion using a spatula. Make a few swirls in the labneh, then drizzle a fairly generous amount of olive oil in the indentations. Sprinkle with za'atar, ganish with the olives in the middle, and serve with bread for dipping.

Mediterranean Tradition

The word *Lebanon* is derived from the word *labneh,* which comes from the Arabic word for milk, *laban. Za'atar* is the Arabic word for a variety of wild thyme. It is also the name of a spice mix, such as what is called for in this recipe, containing the wild thyme, coriander, sesame seeds, Middle Eastern sumac, and sea salt.

Herb and Goat Cheese Vegetable Dip/
Pâte de Fromage de Chèvre aux Herbes Fraîches

Despite its nutritional richness, goat's milk generally has a lower cheese yield than cow's milk, and goat cheeses are less suited to aging. Each different breed of goat and the terrain of the pastures they graze in are responsible for a wide variety of different cheese flavors. This mixture is also fantastic to use as a stuffing for grilled portobello mushrooms.

8 ounces (225 g) soft fresh goat cheese (such as Montrachet)

¼ cup (60 ml) extra-virgin olive oil, divided (preferably unfiltered)

3 tablespoons (45 g) plain yogurt

2 tablespoons (6 g) chopped fresh chives

2 tablespoons (8 g) chopped fresh Italian parsley

1 teaspoon chopped fresh mint

1 teaspoon chopped fresh thyme

½ teaspoon chopped fresh rosemary

Assorted raw vegetables

Yield: 6 servings

Combine the goat cheese, oil, and yogurt in a blender or food processor, and blend until smooth. Transfer to small bowl. Mix in the chives, parsley, mint, thyme, and rosemary. Season dip to taste with salt and pepper. Cover and refrigerate until the dip is cold and flavors blend, 3 hours to overnight, and keep chilled until serving. Serve with vegetables.

Mediterranean Tradition
In addition to the soft, fresh goat cheese most available in the West, goat milk, which is easier for most people to digest, is used by itself and combined with sheep's milk to make yogurt, ricotta, feta, manchego, queso cabrales, and many other kinds of cheese in the southern and eastern portions of the Mediterranean.

Cypriot Greengrocer's Salad with Feta/
Choriatiki Salata

Big, open air vegetable markets are commonplace on the island of Cyprus and in the rest of the region. For people who live too far to reach them, greengrocers usually set up stands or stalls in most neighborhoods. Almost every country in the Mediterranean has this style of salad that is known as Greek salad in the United States. Some cultures may chop the vegetables differently, or add different spices, but the salads themselves are pretty similar. Many cultures also refrain from preparing the dressing in advance, and serve salads with little olive oil and vinegar decanters or lemon slices nearby.

1 head Romaine lettuce, washed, dried, and cut into bite-size pieces

2 ripe tomatoes, diced

1 baby (Persian) cucumber, or ⅓ English cucumber, sliced thinly on the diagonal

¼ pound (115 g) feta, cubed or crumbled

¼ cup Greek olives, pitted

1 yellow onion, sliced into rings

1 small green bell pepper, cut into rings

3 tablespoons (45 ml) red wine vinegar or lemon juice

Unrefined sea salt or salt, to taste

Freshly ground black pepper, to taste

½ cup (120 ml) extra-virgin olive oil (preferably unfiltered)

Yield: 6 servings

Place the lettuce in a large salad bowl. Add the tomatoes and cucumber, and toss to combine.

Scatter the feta, olives, onion, and pepper over the top in an attractive pattern. Pour wine vinegar or lemon juice into a small bowl. Add a pinch of salt and pepper, and slowly pour in the olive oil while whisking vigorously. Once the dressing is emulsified, pour it over the salad and serve immediately.

Mediterranean Tradition
Clever home cooks in the region usually stretch the leftover meat from meals by adding pieces of chicken, beef, veal, and lamb to salads. In Italy, this tradition is called *Insalata del Lunedi*, Monday Salad, because it incorporates the leftover meat from the ritual Sunday gathering.

Spiced Greek Yogurt with Apricots/
Giaoúrti me veríkoka

In Greece, Turkey, and other Balkan countries, yogurt is a popular breakfast and snack. The combination of cinnamon, citrus, and apricots in this recipe make it so sweet and flavorful, that it can double as dessert. I like to serve it in clear martini glasses for an elegant presentation.

2 cups (460 g) full-fat plain Greek yogurt

1 teaspoon pure cinnamon

1 tablespoon (14 g) unsalted butter

1 cup (130 g) dried apricots

⅓ cup (67 g) sugar

Juice and zest of 1 orange

4 teaspoons sliced almonds or chopped, shelled pistachios or walnuts

2 teaspoons honey

Yield: 4 servings

In a medium bowl, combine the yogurt and cinnamon, stirring until incorporated. Heat the butter in a medium skillet over medium-high heat. When the butter melts, add the apricots and toss to coat. Add in the sugar, stir, and reduce heat to medium-low. Allow to cook until the apricots begin to caramelize and plump up, 6 to 8 minutes.

In the meantime, divide the yogurt into 4 serving glasses. When the apricots are ready, deglaze pan with the orange juice. When liquid is almost completely absorbed, stir in orange zest. If sauce doesn't immediately thicken, allow it to simmer, uncovered, over low heat until it is mostly evaporated, 5 to 8 minutes.

Divide the apricot mixture on top of the yogurt in the serving glasses. Top with 1 teaspoon nuts each. Drizzle with ½ teaspoon of honey each, and serve.

Mediterranean Tradition
Yogurt is often used as a substitute for cream among the more health-conscious people in the region. This recipe, even though healthful, has the same smooth and creamy texture as the traditional, yet more fattening, cooked cream desserts.

POULTRY AND EGGS

If you're looking to increase your chicken repertoire, Mediterranean-style chicken dishes are the ultimate in flavor and elegance. Historically, chicken was very expensive throughout the region, and only kings, sultans, and the upper classes could afford it. As a result, the chicken recipes that were created were extravagant and delicious.

The term *poultry* refers to fowl such as chicken, turkey, ducks, and geese. While each of these are eaten in the Mediterranean region, it is chicken that is by far the most popular today, and it is chicken meat that I have focused on in this chapter. The recipes in this collection hail from a wide variety of places in the region and feature roasted, grilled, sautéed, and stewed dishes.

Eggs are another staple in the Mediterranean diet. In the southern European portion of the region they are eaten strictly for dinner, and sometimes lunch, while the North African and Middle Eastern countries also eat them for breakfast. Egg yolks are good sources of omega-3 fats and protein. Although they were traditionally viewed as a meat substitute in many countries because of their lower cost, there are many Mediterranean egg dishes that are so savory, that they are often preferred over meat. For best results, use organic eggs from pasture-raised chickens.

Nutritional Benefits

According to the National Chicken Council, "Chicken consists of high-quality protein and a relatively low amount of fat. In addition, fat in chicken is mostly of the unsaturated type, which protects against heart disease." One 3-ounce (85 g) serving contains just 1 gram of saturated fat and less than 4 grams of total fat, yet is packed with 31 grams of protein, which is more than half of the daily recommended allowance for adult females. Chicken meat contains a significant amount of B vitamins, which aid in metabolism, immune system and blood sugar level maintenance, cell growth, and nerve cell and red blood cell maintenance. It also contains "iron (oxygen transport and cell growth) and zinc (immune system functioning and DNA synthesis)." For these reasons, chicken is a favorite among athletes, dieters, and the health conscious alike.

A popular Mediterranean staple, the egg has gotten a bad nutritional rap during the last few decades when it was linked to increased cholesterol, heart attacks, and strokes. Fortunately, several studies, including one in the *American Journal of Clinical Nutrition,* found no correlation between eggs and heart attack or stroke risks in healthy people. On the contrary, it found that the nutrient choline, found predominantly in egg yolks, may reduce cancer risk.

Egg yolks also contain antioxidants known to prevent macular degeneration. The high protein content in eggs makes you feel full and satisfied longer than other foods, which contributes to weight loss and enables your muscles to repair after a workout. With large eggs containing only 72 calories each and suited to a wide variety of cooking styles, eggs are a natural choice for the health conscious, and budget wary, foodies.

Wine in Moderation

The tenants of the Mediterranean diet allow for wine in moderation. Red wine, in particular, has been shown to have health benefits. For one, it is fermented with its skin, which contains a more concentrated amount of the antioxidant polyphenols and flavonoids. These antioxidants provide cardiovascular protection by preventing blood clotting and reducing arterial plaque. As a bonus, they prevent tumors from growing as well. Most doctors do not advise patients who currently abstain from alcohol to begin drinking specifically for this benefit, because antioxidants can be found in a wide variety of plant-based foods. The Cleveland Clinic recommends two 3½-ounce (104 ml) glasses of red wine for men and one 3½-ounce (104 ml) glass for women per day.

In many portions of the southern and eastern Mediterranean, moderate amounts of local wine are often enjoyed with meals. In North Africa and other areas in the Middle Eastern portion of the region, however, alcohol may be restricted for religious reasons. Instead, locals often enjoy a wide variety of healthful freshly squeezed fruit "cocktails" and herbal tisanes, which have health-promoting properties of their own.

Chicken Skillet-Style *Shwarma* with Tahini Sauce/ *Shwarma Dajaj bil Tahina*

This is my go-to recipe when I'm short on time and have leftover roasted chicken from making Roman *Tavola Calda*– Style Roasted Chicken with Potatoes (opposite), Herb-Marinated Chicken Breasts (page 148), or Jerusalem-Style Chicken (page 150) on hand. *Shwarma* is the rotisserie cooked meat that is shaved and piled high in sandwiches all over Greece, North Africa, and the Middle East. Traditionally, the meat is threaded with layers of fat, topped with tomatoes and peppers, and left to cook slowly for hours. This housewife version is easier and healthier.

2 tablespoons (30 ml) extra-virgin olive oil

1 yellow onion, finely diced

2 red or green bell peppers, trimmed, seeded, and cut into 1-inch (2.5 cm) pieces

2 cups (450 g) shredded cooked chicken meat

1 teaspoon ground coriander

½ teaspoon ground cumin

½ teaspoon unrefined sea salt or salt

¼ teaspoon freshly ground black pepper

2 cups (452 g) diced tomatoes

4 pieces Whole-Wheat Pita Bread (page 19), halved, to serve

1 recipe Tahini Sauce (page 76)

Quick Italian Pickles, to serve (page 60)

Yield: 4 servings

Heat the olive oil in a large skillet over medium heat. Add the onion and peppers and sauté, until lightly golden, about 3 minutes. Add the chicken meat, coriander, cumin, salt, and pepper, and stir. Add the tomatoes and mix well to incorporate. Cover, and cook until peppers are tender, about 5 minutes.

When the chicken mixture is finished cooking, heat the bread. Scoop equal amounts of chicken mixture into the pockets of pita halves. Drizzle Tahini Sauce over the top. Serve warm, with pickled vegetables on the side.

Mediterranean Tradition
Stretching leftover meat with vegetables, herbs, and spices is a great way to pack more nutrients and less fat into your diet.

Roman *Tavola Calda*-Style Roasted Chicken with Potatoes/*Pollo al forno con patate*

Tavola calda means "hot table" in Italian. The term refers to take-out establishments that specialize in rotisserie chickens and ready-to-eat hot dishes such as pizza bianca, potato croquettes, baked pasta, and more—with special twists making them unique to the region they're in. The food served in many of the tavola caldas is so delicious and satisfying, that I often prefer it to that in fine restaurants. In fact, one of my favorite things to do in Rome is to purchase roasted chicken, herb-roasted potatoes, focaccia, and risotto croquettes and take them to a park, such as Villa Borghese, to enjoy.

1 whole chicken (3½ pounds or 1.6 kg), cleaned and rinsed well

¼ cup (60 ml) extra-virgin olive oil

1 teaspoon unrefined sea salt or salt

½ teaspoon freshly ground pepper

1 tablespoon (2 g) finely chopped fresh rosemary

1 head garlic, stem sliced off, left intact

1 lemon, cut in half

1½ pounds (680 g) Yukon gold or other potatoes, peeled and cut into 1-inch (2.5 cm) pieces

Yield: 8 servings

Preheat the oven to 425°F (220°C). Place the chicken in a roasting pan and drizzle olive oil over the chicken, turning to make sure that both the pan and chicken are coated. Season with sea salt, freshly ground pepper, and rosemary by rubbing them into the top and sides of the chicken.

Place garlic and ½ lemon inside the chicken cavity, and squeeze the remaining lemon half over the chicken. Bake, uncovered, for 45 minutes. Carefully (oil tends to splatter), remove the chicken from the oven and scatter potatoes around the edges, turning to coat in olive oil.

Return to the oven to bake for another 45 minutes, or until chicken is done and potatoes are tender. Chicken is done when clear juices run from the thickest part of the thigh after being pierced with a fork, or when internal temperature of meat reaches 165°F (74°C).

Cover the chicken and allow to rest 10 minutes before carving. Discard the garlic and lemon from chicken cavity before serving.

Mediterranean Tradition

Many women in the region, myself included, don't bother roasting one thing at a time. I always make at least two chickens at a time, using leftover chicken to make Chicken Skillet–Style *Shwarma* with Tahini Sauce (opposite), chicken noodle soup, or chicken salad. Other times I roast a chicken and a whole fish, which can be dressed in the same way and needs only one-third of the time to bake. I eat the fish immediately and serve the chicken later in the day or the next—with leftovers on the third day.

Calabrian Chicken, Pepper, Tomato, and Potato Stew/ *Pollo in umido*

In my ancestral homeland of Calabria, Italy, potatoes, peppers, and tomatoes find their way into many recipes. Although they are New World ingredients not available in the region prior to the Columbus trip to America, they now take center stage in most savory dishes, and their addition to a recipe is said to make it Calabrian. Eggs are often served with the trio of vegetables in vegetarian dishes. This piquant stew generally features veal, but I have substituted chicken. Lamb, goat, and beef could also be used. Mediterranean–Style Corn Bread (page 20) or polenta are great accompaniments to this stew.

¼ cup (60 ml) extra-virgin olive oil, divided

1 pound (455 g) boneless chicken breast, cut into 2-inch (5 cm) cubes

1 large onion, roughly chopped

1 large red bell pepper, trimmed, seeded, and cut into 1-inch (2.5 cm) pieces

1 large green bell pepper, trimmed, seeded, and cut into 1-inch (2.5 cm) pieces

2 cloves garlic, minced

2 cups (452 g) diced tomatoes

2 tablespoons (8 g) finely chopped fresh flat-leaf parsley

2 tablespoons (5 g) finely chopped fresh basil

½ teaspoon unrefined sea salt or salt

¼ teaspoon freshly ground black pepper

¼ teaspoon crushed red pepper, or to taste

2 Yukon gold potatoes, peeled, halved, and cut into ¼-inch (6 mm) rounds

Yield: 4 servings

Heat 3 tablespoons (45 ml) of olive oil in a large, heavy-bottomed saucepan over medium heat. Add the chicken and brown on all sides. Remove from the skillet and set on a plate. Add the remaining tablespoon (15 ml) of olive oil, onion, and peppers and sauté, stirring occasionally, until light golden, 3 to 4 minutes. Add garlic and stir. Add the chicken back to the saucepan along with tomatoes, parsley, basil, salt, pepper, and crushed red pepper.

Stir, increase heat to high, and bring to a boil. Reduce heat to medium-low, stir, and cover. Simmer for 20 minutes. Remove the lid, stir, add potatoes, replace the lid, and continue cooking until the meat is cooked through and vegetables are tender, 45 minutes to 1 hour.

Mediterranean Tradition
Stews are a great make-ahead dish, because the meat continues to absorb the liquid in the recipe as it sits, intensifying the flavor. If you would like to make this a day ahead, just bring the hot stew to room temperature before storing it in an airtight container in the refrigerator. Reheat in a saucepan over moderate heat before serving.

Herb-Marinated Chicken Breasts/
Petti di pollo marinati

I make this recipe with whatever fresh herbs I happen to have on hand at least twice a month. It's easy, lean, and delicious. The chicken can also be quickly grilled or broiled. I often slice the leftovers and serve them over a salad made of spinach and arugula, cherry tomatoes, shredded carrots, fresh peas, and corn. This marinade also works well with turkey breasts and firm-fleshed fish.

½ cup (120 ml) fresh lemon juice

¼ cup (60 ml) extra-virgin olive oil

4 cloves garlic, minced

2 tablespoons (5 g) chopped fresh basil

1 tablespoon (4 g) chopped fresh oregano

1 tablespoon (6 g) chopped fresh mint

2 pounds (910 g) chicken breast tenders

½ teaspoon unrefined sea salt or salt

¼ teaspoon freshly ground black pepper

Yield: 4 servings

In a small bowl, whisk the lemon juice, olive oil, garlic, basil, oregano, and mint well to combine. Place the chicken breasts in a large shallow bowl or glass baking pan, and pour dressing over the top.

Cover, place in the refrigerator, and allow to marinate for 1 to 2 hours. Remove from the refrigerator, and season with salt and pepper.

Heat a large, wide skillet over medium-high heat. Using tongs, place chicken tenders evenly in the bottom of the skillet. Pour the remaining marinade over the chicken.

Allow to cook for 3 to 5 minutes each side, or until chicken is golden, juices have been absorbed, and meat is cooked to an internal temperature of 160°F (71°C).

Mediterranean Tradition
You'll find lemon juice used as an ingredient or as a garnish in most fish and poultry recipes in the region. In addition to the taste and moisture that the citrus juice adds to the recipe, lemon's antibacterial properties are coveted for killing bad bacteria in undercooked foods, making them both safe and delicious to eat.

Omelet Provencale

There are two kinds of omelets in Provence: the more commonly known frittata type that is stuffed with Mediterranean ingredients, as well as a *crespeu,* which is a flat omelet that looks like a crêpe stacked and layered with filling. The "cake" consists of three separate flat omelets that are stacked and then "iced" with a simple tapenade mixture. It is accompanied by a ribbon of fresh tomato sauce and a *brandade* crouton. This simple version is easy to make and loaded with fresh Mediterranean flavors.

2 tablespoons (30 ml) extra-virgin olive oil, plus 2 teaspoons for serving

2 zucchini, diced

2 roasted red peppers from a jar, drained and finely chopped

1 clove garlic, finely chopped

¼ cup (12 g) finely chopped chives

8 eggs

½ teaspoon unrefined sea salt or salt

¼ teaspoon freshly ground black pepper

2½ ounces (½ cup, or 38 g) goat cheese

2 tablespoons (5 g) finely chopped fresh basil

4 cups (100 g), mixed field greens, baby spinach, or arugula, to serve

1 teaspoon lemon juice

Yield: 4 servings

Heat 2 tablespoons (30 ml) of the oil in a large skillet over medium heat. Add the zucchini, roasted red pepper, garlic, and chives, then cook gently for about 10 minutes, until softened. Break the eggs into a bowl, whisk lightly and season with salt and pepper. Pour the eggs into the skillet, turn, and swivel to coat. Add knobs of the goat cheese over the top and sprinkle with basil.

Cook until the egg is set and lightly browned underneath, then cover the pan with a plate and invert the omelet onto it. Slide it back into the pan to cook the other side.

To serve, divide 1 cup (25 g) of salad greens onto 4 plates, drizzle with remaining olive oil and lemon juice. Serve a slice of the omelet on the side.

Mediterranean Tradition
Talented Mediterranean cooks can transform any leftover grilled or roasted meat, chicken, fish, vegetables, and even grains and pastas into a tasty omelet.

Jerusalem-Style Chicken with Rice, Golden Raisins, and Pine Nuts/*Dajaj Mashy*

This succulent chicken dish hails from Israel and is accompanied by fragrant basmati rice, which although never grown locally, has been a staple in the Palestinian community for centuries.

For the Chicken:

1 whole roasting chicken (3½ pounds, or 1.6 kg), rinsed, giblets removed, and dried

2 tablespoons (30 ml) extra-virgin olive oil

2 cloves garlic

1 orange, zested and halved

½ teaspoon kosher salt

¼ teaspoon freshly ground pepper

For the Rice:

3 tablespoons (45 ml) extra-virgin olive oil, divided

1 cup (185 g) basmati rice, soaked in water for 20 minutes and drained

1¾ cups (425 ml) boiling water

1 teaspoon allspice

1 teaspoon pure cinnamon

1 teaspoon ground ginger

5 cardamom pods

½ teaspoon unrefined sea salt or salt

¼ cup (35 g) pine nuts

½ cup (70 g) golden raisins, soaked in hot water for 20 minutes and drained

Yield: 4 servings

To make the chicken: Preheat the oven to 425°F (220°C). Place the chicken in a roasting pan greased with olive oil, turning the chicken to coat in oil. Put the garlic cloves and half of the orange in the cavity of the chicken and squeeze the juice from the remaining half over the top and around the base of the pan. Season the chicken with salt and pepper.

Cover with aluminum foil and roast for about 1 hour and 30 minutes (removing foil after 1 hour, basting every 20 minutes or so), or until juices run clear from the thigh of the chicken when pierced, or chicken reaches an internal temperature of 165°F (74°C). (If blood comes out of the thigh from the piercing, the chicken is not yet cooked.)

To make the rice: After the chicken has been roasting for an hour, begin preparing the rice. Heat 2 tablespoons (30 ml) olive oil in a saucepan with a tight-fitting lid over medium heat. Add the rice, boiling water, allspice, cinnamon, ginger, cardamom pods, and salt. Stir to combine and increase heat to high. Bring to a boil, reduce heat to low, and place a paper towel between the pot and the cover to absorb steam as rice cooks.

Cook until all of the liquid is absorbed, 10 to 15 minutes. Remove from heat and allow to sit, covered, for 10 minutes. Remove lid and paper towel and fluff rice with a fork. Taste and adjust seasonings if necessary.

Heat the remaining 1 tablespoon (15 ml) olive oil in a small skillet over medium heat, and add the pine nuts and raisins. Toast until they start to turn golden and the nuts begin to release their aroma, 3 to 5 minutes. Scatter over rice.

When the chicken is finished roasting, remove from the oven and cover with aluminum foil. Allow to rest for 10 minutes, carve, drizzle with pan juices, and serve hot with rice. Sprinkle orange zest over the top.

Mediterranean Tradition

Orange zest is a popular addition to many Middle Eastern rice pilafs. Just one teaspoon of orange peel per week is has been shown to reduce skin cancer risk by 30 percent.

Israeli *Shakshouka*-Style Eggs/*Shakshouka*

This dish is of Tunisian, Algerian, Moroccan, and Libyan origin, and is nowadays extremely popular in Israel. Served for breakfast, lunch, or dinner, traditionally in a cast iron pan—this is one of the tastiest, easiest, and most economical dishes around.

2 tablespoons (30 ml) extra-virgin olive oil

2 tablespoons (30 g) harissa sauce (see page 184)

2 tablespoons (32 g) tomato paste

1 teaspoon smoked paprika

1 yellow onion, diced

2 large red peppers, trimmed, seeded, and cut into small pieces

3 cups (678 g) chopped very ripe tomatoes

6 large organic eggs

½ cup (115 g) Labneh (page 136), or plain Greek yogurt

4 pieces Whole-Wheat Pita Bread (page 19) or other pita, warmed, for serving

Yield: 4 servings

Heat the olive oil in a large skillet over medium heat. Add the harissa, tomato paste, paprika, onion and peppers. Stir well to combine and allow to cook until peppers are tender, 5 to 7 minutes. Add the tomatoes, stir, and increase heat to high. When mixture begins to boil, reduce heat to low and simmer until sauce thickens, about 10 minutes. Taste and adjust seasoning.

Make 6 wells in the sauce. Break eggs into the wells. Using a fork, gently swirl the egg whites into the sauce. Simmer, uncovered, until the egg whites are set but the egg yolks are not yet hard, 6 to 8 minutes. Remove from heat and allow to set for a few minutes before serving. Serve with labneh or yogurt and hot pita bread.

Mediterranean Tradition

Eggs are enjoyed with peppers, tomatoes, and potatoes all over the region. To make an even quicker version of this dish, combine leftover roasted or grilled vegetables with tomatoes in a skillet heated with a tablespoon (15 ml) of olive oil. Break in eggs and scramble.

Tunisian Egg, Tuna, and Tomato Sandwiches/ *Casse-Croûte Tunisien*

A quarter of the world's olive oil supply comes from the North African nation of Tunisia. Boasting a beautiful landscape and coastline along with a cosmopolitan culture, Tunisia's delicious cuisine, a height of gourmet creativity since Medieval times, often gets overshadowed by that of neighboring Morocco. One of Tunisia's most popular street foods are *brek,* a deep-fried turnover filled with tuna and vegetables left over from the Ottoman era, and Casse-Croûte—sandwiches filled with similar ingredients.

¼ cup (60 ml) extra-virgin olive oil

2 cloves garlic, minced

½ small yellow onion, minced

½ small green bell pepper, stemmed, seeded, and minced

1 medium ripe tomato, diced

Unrefined sea salt or salt, to taste

Freshly ground black pepper, to taste

4 small hero or sandwich rolls

1 small English cucumber, thinly sliced

1 medium ripe tomato, thinly sliced

9 or 10 ounces (255 to 283 g) tuna in olive oil, drained well

2 hardboiled eggs, sliced into quarters

½ cup (50 g) pitted black olives

4 jarred pepperoncini peppers, drained, stemmed, and halved lengthwise

½ cup (120 g) harissa (see page 184) or other hot sauce

Yield: 4 servings

Heat the olive oil in a large skillet over medium-high heat. Add the garlic, onion, pepper, and diced tomato, and cook, stirring, until soft, about 6 minutes. Season with salt and pepper, and set aside.

Split the rolls horizontally, leaving them intact on one side. Divide the tomato sauce among rolls, top with cucumber, and sliced tomato, and then tuna; top with eggs, olives, and pepperoncini. Drizzle the top of each with harissa and serve.

Mediterranean Tradition
The powerful, high-protein duo of tuna and eggs is a classic combination throughout the region. For example, in Italy, they are tossed into salads with white beans; in Provence, they are star elements in the *salade niçoise*; and in North Africa, they're popular additions to savory pies. Try incorporating them into some of your favorite dishes to boost their nutritional benefits.

Seasonal Italian Frittata/*Frittata stagionale*

Frittate, as they are called in Italian, can be downsized into mini portions for the perfect appetizer, or served in large slices for a hearty, vegetarian breakfast, lunch, and dinner. When CNN.com asked me to prepare my ultimate menu for Prince William's 2011 wedding, I included bite-size frittatas as part of the appetizer course. The ingredients in this classic Italian version can be found year-round in most supermarkets. Try swapping out the zucchini and potatoes for artichokes and asparagus in spring, tomatoes and eggplant in summer, and fennel and roasted peppers in the fall.

¼ cup (60 ml) extra-virgin olive oil

½ medium yellow onion, cut into very thin slices

1 pint (175 g) shitake mushrooms, stemmed and cut into very thin (⅛-inch, or 3 mm) slices

1 large or 2 small leeks, white and light green parts rinsed and finely chopped

8 basil leaves, hand torn

6 large eggs, beaten in a bowl until foamy

¼ cup (30 g) grated Pecorino Romano

1 teaspoon unrefined sea salt or salt

Yield: 4 servings

Preheat the oven to 350°F (180°C). Heat the oil in a large, wide, ovenproof skillet over medium-high heat.

Add the onion and sauté, stirring occasionally, until softened and golden, 4 minutes. Add mushrooms and brown them, 4 minutes. Add the leeks, stir, and cook for another 4 minutes.

Add the basil leaves, beaten eggs, Pecorino Romano, and salt. Mix well and reduce heat to medium-low. Cook, undisturbed, for 4 to 5 minutes, or until the eggs are cooked through.

Finish off the frittata by putting the skillet in the oven until the frittata top is golden and the eggs are set. Cut into 4 pieces and serve.

Mediterranean Tradition
Frittatas and other omelets are usually served as light dinners along with salad in Mediterranean countries.

Meats & Sweets: Mediterranean Indulgences

Meat and sweets are paired together in this chapter to emphasize that they should be eaten sparingly, as the Mediterranean Diet Pyramid suggests. These two types of foods are worlds apart, culinarily speaking, but their high-fat content makes them an indulgence, not a daily ritual. To keep with a healthful lifestyle, the types of meat dishes and sweets in this book are rather healthful compared with what is available at cafés, restaurants, and on store shelves.

To many, the word *Mediterranean* with the terms *food* or *cuisine* calls to mind an image of lamb roasting on a spit. For many people in other places, slow-roasted lamb is symbolic of many countries in the region, and different from the culinary traditions of their own cultures. One reason lamb is so traditional, is because it was eaten only on occasion, usually in the spring, when Easter, Passover, a Muslim holiday, or a wedding was celebrated. This tradition dates back to Bedouin times when nomadic tribes had to travel with their livestock. They refrained from killing them for meat because it would cut off their milk supply that was needed to make the yogurt and cheeses that people relied on for daily sustenance. As a result, whenever meat was served, it was to honor a guest. Newcomers to the region were treated to as much meat as possible out of respect.

The fact that daily indulgence in meat is not the norm is what has made the Mediterranean diet so successful. Because meat is eaten infrequently, meat-based recipes tend to be decadent, slow-cooked, and delicious. Save these recipes for a special occasion or time when you don't have to hurry in the kitchen. While none of them are complicated, they do take a little more time than most weeknight recipes. The warm, herbal, and spicy aromas wafting in the air alone will prove that your patience has paid off.

MEATS

Lamb, goat, veal, and beef are enjoyed throughout the Mediterranean. In my years as a cooking instructor, I was amazed to find out how many people had aversions to lamb, goat, and veal—all for various reasons. Yet, these meats offer great flavor and nutrition, as well as blank culinary canvases to build upon.

Goats are known for their hardiness and ability to adapt to difficult conditions. Domesticated in Syria around 8,000 BCE, goats underwent an evolution that significantly changed their morphology before goat farming was introduced to Europe and then the rest of the world. As the animals took to various terrains, different types of breeds developed (there are currently more than 300 varieties worldwide). Sheep and goats were not raised specifically for their meat, as they are in many places today. Instead, early nomadic cultures traveled with the animals for their milk, which would be transformed into yogurt and cheese; slaughtering one to eat its meat was viewed as wasteful. Meat was usually only served in order to honor a guest visiting the tribe, or for a holiday or wedding. Over the thousands of years that have passed, the notion of meat being special has become deeply interwoven into the culture of the Middle Eastern portion of the Mediterranean.

The popularity of lamb meat in the Mediterranean didn't come by accident. In addition to its popularity in antiquity, the monotheistic faiths also helped to make it more widely appreciated. The symbolism of lamb in the Judeo-Christian-Islamic faiths made it even more popular—and since sheep give birth in the late winter, it became the meat of choice for Passover, Easter, weddings, and other spring holidays. Lamb meat is easy to prepare, works well in a wide variety of culinary applications, and is healthful.

Nutritional Benefits

There are many reasons to love goat. First of all, goat meat is easily digestible by the body. It is also lean, easy to prepare, and lends itself to a wide variety of preparations and cuisines. Goats are also good for the environment thanks to their eco-friendly grazing patterns. While offering a significant amount of protein, goat meat is the leanest of all meats (other than ostrich), has the lowest amount of cholesterol, and offers generous amounts of iron and other nutrients.

I grew up eating lamb as part of the Greek Easter celebrations. According to the Tri-Lamb Group, on average, a 3-ounce (85 g) serving of lamb is lean—about 175 calories. Lean cuts include the leg, loin, and rack. Lamb provides vitamins and minerals and is an excellent source of protein, which helps keep hunger at bay, preserves lean body mass, and regulates blood sugar. A 3-ounce (85 g) serving has 23 grams of protein—nearly half of the daily recommended needs. The same serving size also offers a good dose of heart-healthy monounsaturated fat and almost five times the amount of omega-3 fatty acids as found in beef.

Both veal and beef have similar amounts of protein (approximately 30 grams per 3 ounces (85 g) of meat). Beef has slightly less fat, cholesterol, and calories than veal, but both meats are good sources of B vitamins that are needed for energy. They are also significant sources of riboflavin, niacin, and pantothenic acid.

Both beef and veal contain approximately one-quarter of the daily recommended value of zinc. Red meat, in general, offers more B_{12}, iron, and zinc than white meat as well as a higher amount of healthful fatty acids. Goat, sheep, and beef fat (as well as that of other ruminants) contains about equal parts saturated and monounsaturated fat with only a small quantity of polyunsaturated fat.

The Mediterranean diet recommends eating less than 1 pound (455 g) of red meat per month—which breaks down to approximately one 4-ounce (115 g) serving per week. While the traditional eating patterns in the Mediterranean region don't prescribe eating meat daily, when it is eaten, delicious, high-quality, fresh meat is enjoyed. Eating meat sparingly seems only to enhance its image as the ultimate demonstration of hospitality in the region. In most places it is considered disrespectful to serve guests a vegetarian meal. The lack of meat on the table means that you are too poor to afford it, or that you do not think your guest is worthy of receiving it. These recipes will show any guest that he or she is indeed worth it.

I realize that many people might be alarmed at my decision to combine meats and sweets in the same chapter, but I can assure you it's for good reason.

Middle Eastern Lamb and Okra Stew/
Lahma Dani bil Bamya

Often made in earthenware brams, Middle Eastern stews are the epitome of home cooking. Traditionally served with rice, the combination of slowly roasted meat and vegetables produce a rich, indulgent flavor that makes one forget how nutritious the dish is. This is a great stew to make in advance, because it tastes even better the next day.

2 tablespoons (30 ml) extra-virgin olive oil

1 large yellow onion, chopped

2 pounds (910 g) boneless lamb leg or shoulder, cut into 1 to 2-inch (2.5 to 5 cm) cubes

1 teaspoon dried coriander

¼ teaspoon ground cumin

¼ teaspoon ground cinnamon

¼ teaspoon ground nutmeg

¼ teaspoon paprika

2 cups (475 ml) Chicken or Beef Stock (see page 183)

¼ teaspoon unrefined sea salt or salt, or to taste

Freshly ground black pepper, to taste

1 cup (250 g) tomato purée

1 pound (455 g) fresh okra, stems removed and cut into ¼-inch (6 mm) rounds or frozen chopped okra, thawed

Juice of 1 lemon or lime

Yield: 6 servings

Heat the olive oil in a large saucepan over medium heat. Add the onion and stir. When the onion turns translucent, about 5 minutes, add the lamb cubes and brown on all sides. Add the coriander, cumin, cinnamon, nutmeg, paprika, stock, salt, and pepper. Increase heat to high and bring to a boil.

Reduce heat to low, cover, and simmer for 1 hour, stirring occasionally.

Add the tomato purée and okra, stir and cover. Cook for another 30 minutes, until the lamb and okra are tender. Taste and adjust salt and pepper, if necessary. Stir in lemon or lime juice. Serve warm.

Mediterranean Tradition

The Spanish Umayyad Prince Abd al Rahman brought okra to Europe from Egypt in the ninth century. When choosing okra, choose firm bright green ones. A soft texture and discoloration are signs that they are beyond their peak. Baby okra can be left whole and used in this recipe as well. If you're not a fan of okra, you could substitute green beans, or any other seasonal vegetable instead.

Sicilian Stuffed Veal Roast/*Arrosto di vitello*

Traditionally, roasts were made during cooler periods in the Mediterranean because the oven played a key role in warming the home before centralized heating was common. Making roasts on the weekly day of rest is a tradition throughout the Mediterranean region. In addition to their great taste, they require little effort to make and are capable of feeding large crowds. Even if you're cooking for 1 or 2 people, roasts are still worth making. You can eat them as a traditional meal, use leftovers in salads, sandwiches, and pasta dishes, and freeze the rest for a later date. Note that you will need butcher's twine to complete this recipe.

¼ cup (60 ml) extra-virgin olive oil, divided

1 bunch fresh flat-leaf Italian parsley

10 ounces (280 g) pitted green olives, Sicilian Colossal variety, if possible

¼ cup (35 g) pine nuts

2 cloves garlic

¼ cup (35 g) raisins

Zest of 1 orange

1 boneless breast of veal roast (3 pounds, or 1.4 kg)

1 teaspoon unrefined sea salt or salt

½ teaspoon freshly ground black pepper

3 carrots, chopped

3 ribs celery, chopped

1 medium yellow onion, chopped

2 cups (475 ml) homemade or low-sodium Chicken Stock (see page 183)

1 cup (226 g) chopped or diced no-salt-added tomatoes

Yield: 4 servings

Preheat the oven to 400°F (200°C). Combine 2 tablespoons (30 ml) of olive oil, parsley, olives, pine nuts, and garlic cloves in a food processor, and pulse on and off until you obtain a paste. Remove lid and blade and stir in raisins and orange zest.

Season both sides of the veal with salt and pepper. Spread the stuffing paste evenly over the surface of the veal, generously covering it. Re-roll the roast and tie it with butcher's twine just tightly enough to secure; don't tie too tightly or the filling will ooze out.

Heat the remaining 2 tablespoons (30 ml) of olive oil in an ovenproof casserole or pan over medium-high heat. Add the veal roast and brown on all sides. Add the carrots, celery, and onion, and stir. Add the chicken stock, and tomatoes to the pan. Stir, remove from heat and cover.

Place the roast in the oven and cook for 2 hours or until veal is tender. When the veal is ready, remove from the oven, and carefully place the meat on a cutting board and allow to rest for 10 minutes. To serve, slice the veal and pour sauce over the top.

Mediterranean Tradition
Veal is adored by many in the Mediterranean region. The most prized of all is milk-fed veal, which is loved for its tender, succulent flavor. Check with your local butcher or supermarket before making a trip, as veal often needs to be special ordered.

Southern Italian Goat and Herb Stew/*Pignata di Capra*

This savory stew has been prepared in Basilicata, Calabria, Puglia, and Abruzzo since antiquity. A true testament of farm-to-table cuisine, it was generally made with male goats or mutton because their fibrous meat was too tough to be prepared other ways. This dish can be made in its original version containing only a handful of ingredients, or in a more decadent version that incorporates the freshest seasonal vegetables, aged cheese, sausage, herbs, and spices.

¼ cup (60 ml) extra-virgin olive oil

½ pound (225 g) yellow onions, peeled and roughly chopped

½ pound (225 g) carrots, peeled and cut into 2-inch (5 cm) pieces

1 rib celery, cut into 1-inch (2.5 cm) pieces

6 cloves garlic, sliced

2½ pounds (1 kg) goat (other meat such as beef, veal, or lamb) or cubed, from the thigh or shoulder, about 1½ inches (4 cm) each

1 teaspoon unrefined sea salt or salt

3 sprigs fresh rosemary, leaves finely chopped

1 bunch fresh thyme, finely chopped

4 cups (950 ml) water or Beef Stock (page 183)

1 bay leaf

1 pound (455 g) Yukon gold potatoes, scrubbed, peeled, and cut into 2-inch (5 cm) pieces

1 cup (226 g) crushed peeled tomatoes

¼ teaspoon crushed red chile pepper

Yield: 6 servings

Heat the olive oil in a large, heavy-bottomed saucepan or Dutch oven over medium-high heat.

Add the onions, carrot, and celery, and turn to coat in oil. Reduce heat to medium-low and sauté until tender, about 5 minutes. Add the garlic, stir, and cook for 1 minute, or until it releases its aroma.

Add the goat meat (or other meat) and cook 3 to 5 minutes, until browned on all sides.

Season with salt and stir in rosemary and thyme. Add the stock and bay leaf. Increase heat to high and bring to a boil. Stir, reduce heat to low, cover, and simmer for 2½ hours, stirring occasionally.

Add the potatoes, tomatoes, and crushed red chile pepper. Stir, and cover. Cook for another hour, or until the meat is very tender. Taste and adjust seasonings, and remove the bay leaf before serving.

Mediterranean Tradition
In 2014, Chef Luigi Diotauti and I presented a program and created a podcast called "The Goodness of Goat" for the International Association of Culinary Professionals annual conference in Chicago. We continue to promote goat through our joint efforts and consider it "the meat of the future." Even so, it still can be a challenge to find. Call local ethnic butchers to special order, if possible. Goat meat can replace lamb or beef in many recipes. Try it grilled, roasted, or braised for a delicious and low-fat meat entrée.

Herb-Roasted Leg of Lamb/*Lahma dani fihl forn*

Succulent, juicy lamb meat is always served well-done in the Mediterranean region. A symbol of hospitality for millennia, this is an excellent celebratory dish that your guests will appreciate.

1 leg of lamb (5 pounds, or 2.3 kg)

1 head of garlic, peeled

½ teaspoon unrefined sea salt or salt, plus to taste

¼ teaspoon freshly ground black pepper, plus to taste

2 cups (475 ml) Chicken Stock (see page 183), or water, divided

Juice of 1 lemon

2 large yellow onions, sliced into rings

2 tablespoons (30 ml) extra-virgin olive oil

2 large tomatoes, chopped, or ½ cup (113 g) chopped canned tomatoes

2 cinnamon sticks

Yield: 10 servings

Preheat the oven to 350°F (180°C). With a paring knife, make 1-inch (2.5 cm) slits in various places around leg of lamb. Sliver garlic cloves and insert them into the slits in the lamb. Massage ½ teaspoon salt and ¼ teaspoon pepper into the leg of the lamb. Place lamb in a large roasting pan. Pour 1 cup (235 ml) of the chicken stock or water into the pan. Bake for 1 hour, uncovered, basting every 20 minutes.

Pour lemon juice over the lamb. Place the onion rings over the top and drizzle olive oil over the onions. Scatter the tomatoes around the sides of the pan. Add the cinnamon sticks and remaining 1 cup of stock to the pan. Return to the oven and bake, uncovered, an additional 2 hours, basting every 20 minutes, until lamb falls off the bone.

Remove from the oven and cover the pan with lid or aluminum foil. Allow the lamb meat to stand at room temperature for 10 minutes before carving. Remove and discard cinnamon sticks. Place the lamb on a serving platter and carve. Serve warm, with tomatoes and onions spooned over the top.

Mediterranean Tradition

This type of roast—once synonymous with Easter, weddings, and important feasts—is now often enjoyed at weekly family gatherings. For an easy side dish, try adding potatoes or other root vegetables; fennel, peppers, and carrots could all be added during the last hour of cooking. Leftover lamb meat tastes great in salads, as filling for stuffed pastas, and in place of chicken in Chicken Skillet–Style *Shwarma* with Tahini Sauce (page 144).

Corsican-Style Garlic-Laced Beef Stew with Peppers/ *Daube de boeuf corse*

Although meat and pasta dishes are generally served as separate courses in Italy, there are a handful of hearty, rustic dishes such as this that fuse the first and second courses in one glorious plate. The incredibly beautiful Mediterranean island of Corsica was ruled by Italy until the mid-nineteenth century, when it became part of France. By combining both Italian and French country-style cooking with local specialties, Corsica developed a cuisine as awe inspiring as its scenery. In this recipe, lamb, or goat meat could be substituted.

1 pound (455 g) beef stew cubes (2-inch, or 5 cm, pieces)

10 cloves garlic, sliced into thin slivers

1½ teaspoons unrefined sea salt or salt, divided

¾ teaspoon freshly ground black pepper, divided

3 tablespoons (30 ml) olive oil

2 yellow onions, thinly sliced

½ cup (120 ml) dry red wine

2 whole green bell peppers, cut into 4-inch (10 cm) strips

2 cups (452 g) diced tomatoes

1 cinnamon stick

1 bay leaf

1 teaspoon smoked paprika

1 pound (455 g) large tubular pasta such as *maccheroni* or quinoa pasta macaroni, prepared according to package directions

⅔ cup (79 g) freshly grated Pecorino Romano

Yield: 4 servings

With a sharp knife, make slits into each piece of beef and stuff with a few of the garlic slivers. Season the meat with 1 teaspoon salt and ½ teaspoon pepper.

Heat the oil in a Dutch oven or large, heavy-bottomed saucepan over medium heat. Working in batches, brown the meat on all sides. Transfer to a plate. Add the sliced onions to the pan and sauté until lightly golden and soft, about 5 minutes.

Pour the wine into the pan, and stir in the meat. Increase heat to high and cook, stirring often, until wine almost disappears, 3 to 5 minutes. Add the peppers and any remaining garlic to the pan and turn to coat. Add the tomatoes, cinnamon, bay leaf, paprika, remaining salt and pepper, and stir to combine.

Cover, reduce heat to medium-low, and simmer for 2 to 2½ hours, or until the meat is extremely tender, stirring every half hour, and adding water ½ cup (120 ml) at a time if sauce seems too dry. Remove the bay leaf and cinnamon stick.

To serve, stir a little bit of the sauce into the pasta. Spoon the pasta onto a large serving platter, and ladle the remaining meat and sauce over the top. Garnish with the Pecorino Romano.

Mediterranean Tradition
Lacing meat with garlic and simmering it slowly in liquid was a cooking method originally developed to tenderize tough, less expensive meat cuts. The texture and flavor that it produces, however, rival even the choicest cuts.

Greek Cinnamon-Scented Lamb Meatballs/ *Soudsoukakia*

The Greek word for these long, croquette-shaped meatballs is *Keftedes*. When slowly simmered in tomato sauce, they become *Soudsoukakia*. This recipe tastes delicious both ways. If you'd like to serve the meatballs without the sauce, simply grill or broil them until you achieve the desired doneness. I sometimes serve them plain the first night and then simmer the leftovers in tomato sauce the next day. The sweet, spicy aromas of the tomato sauce are so delicious that they entice even those who don't generally eat lamb meat. You can use veal, turkey, or beef in this recipe as well.

For the Meatballs:

2 pounds (910 g) ground lamb

1 medium yellow onion, quartered

6 cloves garlic, roughly chopped

1 teaspoon ground cumin

1 teaspoon pure cinnamon

½ teaspoon unrefined sea salt or salt

¼ teaspoon freshly ground black pepper

For the Sauce:

1 tablespoon (15 ml) olive oil

1 small onion, finely chopped

4 cloves garlic, minced

4 cups (1 kg) tomato purée

Unrefined sea salt or salt

Freshly ground pepper

1 cinnamon stick

Yield: 6 servings (about 6 cups)

To make the meatballs: Preheat the broiler. Combine the lamb, onion, garlic, cumin, cinnamon, salt, and pepper in a food processor. Pulse on and off until mixture turns into a rough paste. Turn the mixture out onto a work surface. Form 12 meatballs that are about 2½-inches (6.5 cm) long and 1-inch (2.5 cm) wide in the center and tapering off to blunted tips at each end.

Place the meatballs on a baking sheet. Brown for about 10 minutes per side, turning after every 2 to 3 minutes. Turn and brown until they are golden on the outside and cooked through on the inside. If the meatballs are finished before the rest of the meal, wrap them in tin foil until needed.

To make the sauce: Heat the olive oil in a saucepan over medium heat. Add the onion and sauté until lightly golden and tender, 3 to 5 minutes. Stir in the garlic and cook until it releases its aroma, about 1 minute. Add the tomato purée, salt and pepper to taste, and cinnamon stick. Bring the mixture to a boil and reduce heat to low.

Gently add the meatballs to the sauce and turn to coat. Cover, reduce heat to low, and simmer until sauce has thickened by half, about 15 to 20 minutes.

Mediterranean Tradition

These meatballs are often threaded onto skewers and grilled, like kabobs. While shaping them, be sure to keep a bowl of water next to you to wet your hands, which helps to make the meatballs adhere to the skewers. Pierce skewer through the middle of them. Thread three *koftedes* onto each skewer. Shape them around the skewer so that it doesn't break or fall off during cooking. Do not crowd or push them too close together. Grill over a medium-high heat, turning often, until cooked to an internal temperature of about 160°F (71°C).

SWEETS

Sweets are not eaten on a daily basis in the traditional Mediterranean diet. Although they are available in massive quantities everywhere, locals usually reserve them for weekly family gatherings and special occasions. Sweets were considered a luxury since the days of the ancient Egyptians when the cost of sugar and finely milled wheat was so high that they could not be afforded by commoners. Instead, fruit, honey, and nuts were the desserts of the day.

It is said that Cleopatra used sugar extravagantly, even though it was extremely expensive, because the Egyptians had just been introduced to the sugar cane crop via the Persians. Sugar was not widely available for all classes in Europe until the nineteenth century. Even though it was available, its cost was prohibitive, as was that of finely milled flour, butter, eggs, and other baking ingredients. As a result, the tradition of eating desserts after a meal was not upheld by the masses. Instead, people ate fresh, seasonal fruit after their meals, just as they do today. Whenever you find yourself eating in someone's home for dinner in the South of France, Italy, Greece, Egypt, or practically any other country in the region, large trays of fruit will be served after a meal.

Throughout history in the Mediterranean region, cakes were served on special occasions such as religious holidays, name days, and as offerings (first to the gods and later to the priests and religious officials). Cakes themselves date back to ancient Egypt. Old Kingdom (2700–2600 BC) tomb scenes depict bread being shaped and produced in mass quantities. Ramses II's tomb revealed pictures of elegant pastries, cakes, and pies being made in bakeries which catered specifically to royalty. The Roman philosopher Cato wrote about cakes after Romans took control of Egypt and gained access to wheat and sugar. Ancient Greek cakes were made of honey and fruits. Typically, the Roman and Greek cakes were used as offerings to the gods. Byzantine desserts (fourth- to fourteenth-century CE), served at the imperial palace, were often cakes made of honey and nuts and enhanced with spices traded from distant lands.

In Medieval England the terms bread and cake were synonymous—a cake usually referred to small bread. During the renaissance in Italy, baking really took off and caused both English and French to import Italian pastry chefs to work for them. By the seventeenth century, baking pans consisted of round rings which were placed on flat surfaces. The round symbol has been used since antiquity as a symbol of the life cycle itself. Many artisan bakers in the region create sweat breads, honey/nut/spice cakes, and rustic cookies in special types of bakeries (often called ovens in their native tongues.) These sweets use quality ingredients and traditional methods and differ greatly from the super sweet, glazed confections of today.

Nutritional Benefits

In Medieval Iraq, desserts were believed to be good for you thanks to the Galenic humoral theory, which divided foods into the wet, dry, hot, and cold categories. Galen was an ancient Greek physician, surgeon, and philosopher in the Roman Empire whose work preceded that of Hippocrates. His theories dominated western medical thought for approximately 1,400 years.

There are still fourteen Arabic cookbooks available from that time period that detail, among other decadent things, glorious desserts. The wealthy empires and caliphates of the day prized themselves on their desserts, and the Ottomans of Turkey were no exception. With their enormous wealth, they heightened a simple Lenten fasting food into the baklava we know today, invented or re-interpreted scores of Mediterranean desserts, and during their rule in various places, influenced the local culinary culture.

While it is no longer common to find medical doctors or diet plans promoting the consumption of sweets, they are permitted for the sole purpose of indulgence. It is believed that if you occasionally allow yourself a small pleasure, that you will be able to adhere to a healthy diet plan the majority of the time. Diets that restrict sweets completely are harder to follow, and their followers tend to be less successful over long periods of time. The desserts chosen in this chapter were included because of their healthful ingredients and delicious taste.

Raspberry Citrus Clafoutis/*Clafoutis aux framboise*

This is one of my favorite pantry desserts—a sweet that you can whip up in minutes with just a few simple ingredients. A *clafoutis* is a typical home-style French dessert resembling a thick cakey baked custard, sometimes called a French flan. Its name (sometimes spelled *clafouti*) originates from the French verb *claufir*, which means "to attach with nails." This is a wonderful recipe to have on hand because it's simple enough for novices to make yet impressive enough for experts to savor. Blueberries, cherries, pears, apples, plums, and prunes could all be used instead of raspberries.

¼ teaspoon unsalted butter

5 tablespoons (65 g) sugar, divided

2 extra-large eggs

½ cup (63 g) unbleached, all-purpose flour or finely ground almond powder

1 cup (235 ml) heavy cream

1 teaspoon pure vanilla extract

1 teaspoon orange zest

1 teaspoon orange blossom water (see page 185) or almond extract

Pinch of unrefined sea salt or salt

1 cup (125 g) raspberries

Confectioners' sugar, for dusting

Yield: 4 servings

Preheat the oven to 375°F (190°C). Butter an 8-inch (20 cm) baking dish. Sprinkle 2 tablespoons (26 g) granulated sugar over the bottom. Beat the eggs and the remaining 3 tablespoons (39 g) sugar in the bowl of an electric mixer fitted with the paddle attachment on medium-high speed, until light and fluffy, about 3 minutes. With mixer running on low speed, add in the flour, cream, vanilla extract, orange zest, orange blossom water or almond extract, and salt.

Add the raspberries to the bottom of the baking dish, turn to coat in sugar, and pour the batter over the top. Bake for 15 to 20 minutes, until the top is golden and custard is set. Serve warm, sprinkled with confectioners' sugar.

Mediterranean Tradition
This is the type of dessert that French housewives would traditionally whip up without a recipe. Throughout the region, homey, satisfying desserts are made that way. It's a great idea to remember the general formula of your favorite baking recipes—as well as how they look and smell while baking so that they can be recreated anytime, anywhere.

Almond-Stuffed Figs in Chocolate Sauce/
Ficchi al Cioccolato

Ounce per ounce, figs contain more nutrients than any other fruit, and nutrient-rich almonds are considered one of the world's healthiest foods. Antioxidant rich dark chocolate, which should be eaten in extreme moderation for its fat content, is known to balance blood sugar levels in people with diabetes when eaten in small quantities. If I had to pick only one dessert to enjoy in life, this would be it—not for its health boosting virtues, but because of its combination of sensual textures and tastes. It's very common in my ancestral homeland of Calabria, Italy, which is known for its prized figs.

20 fresh, ripe figs or good-quality dried white figs

¼ cup (27 g) slivered almonds

Zest of 1 orange, or ¼ cup candied citrus peel

1 teaspoon ground pure cinnamon

½ teaspoon ground cloves

4 ounces (115 g) good-quality dark chocolate

Yield: 4 servings

Preheat the oven to 350°F (180°C). Line two baking sheets with parchment paper.

With the fig upright, make an incision halfway down to the bottom, and open with your fingers. In a small bowl, combine the almonds, orange zest or peel, cinnamon, and cloves. Stuff each of the figs with the filling. Press the figs closed and place them an inch (2.5 cm) apart on one baking sheet. Bake until slightly softened and darkened, 5 to 8 minutes.

Place the chocolate in the top of a double boiler over low heat. Heat, stirring constantly, just until chocolate is melted, 2 to 3 minutes.

Remove the figs from the oven, and using tongs, or holding figs by the stem, dip them quickly into the warm chocolate. Place on the second baking sheet and allow to cool. Store in an airtight container in the refrigerator. Allow to stand at room temperature for at least 20 minutes before serving.

Mediterranean Tradition
This recipe is usually reserved for Christmas and New Year's Day, but I like to make them as edible gifts for my loved ones throughout the year. Figs, which are often linked to sexuality in Mediterranean folklore, have actually been proven to help men overcome sterility in modern times due to their zinc content.

Seasonal Italian Fruit Torte/*Torta di frutta stagionale*

This traditional European cake is a favorite of my family. Light and airy, it's a great way to start the day or end a meal, and can be made with a variety of fruits. This cake is perfect to bring to a potluck or give as a hostess gift. Since it can be frozen for up to a month, I usually make two at a time, one for now, and one to give away whenever the occasion calls. If you're not planning on finishing it the same day, make sure to refrigerate it so that it won't spoil.

6 tablespoons (98 g) unsalted butter, at room temperature, plus more for pan

⅓ cup, plus 1 tablespoon (80 g) sugar

2 large eggs, separated

1 cup (125 g) unbleached, all-purpose flour or almond flour, plus extra for pan

2 ½ teaspoons baking powder

¼ cup (60 ml) heavy cream

2 teaspoons anise or almond extract

2 teaspoons vanilla extract

2 ripe plums, apricots, or nectarines, peeled, pitted, and sliced

or

1 cup (145 g) blueberries

Confectioners' sugar for dusting

Yield: 8 servings

Preheat the oven to 350°F (180°C).

Butter a 9-inch (23 cm) tart pan with a removable bottom. Add a round of parchment, butter the parchment, then flour it.

Place 6 tablespoons (84 g) of butter and ⅓ cup (67 g) sugar in the bowl of an electric mixer fitted with the paddle attachment. Beat together on low speed until smooth and fluffy. Add the egg yolks and beat well until combined.

In a small bowl, stir together the flour and the baking powder. In another small bowl, stir together the cream, ¼ cup (60 ml) water, anise or almond extract, and vanilla extract. Stir the mixtures into the butter mixture by alternating the flour mixture with the cream mixture—adding one-third of each at a time until they are used up.

In a clean bowl fitted to an electric mixer using a whisk attachment, whip the egg whites until stiff peaks form. If the eggs are not stiff enough, the cake will not rise properly.

Using a rubber spatula, gently fold the beaten egg whites into the batter to eliminate all of the white and break up any lumps. Then stir once in the opposite direction to make sure that all white has been incorporated.

Pour the batter into the prepared tart pan and level the surface. Arrange the plums or other fruit in a circle pattern on top of the batter. Sprinkle the remaining tablespoon (13 g) of sugar on top of the fruit.

Bake until a toothpick inserted into the middle of the cake comes out clean and cake begins to pull away from the sides of the pan, 35 to 40 minutes.

Transfer to a cooling rack. Allow cake to cool for at least 30 minutes.

Invert onto a cooling rack and remove sides of pan, then bottom and parchment paper. Turn over to cool completely.

Invert the cake onto another plate and then back over onto a serving platter. Dust with confectioners' sugar. Serve at room temperature.

Mediterranean Tradition
All across the northern Mediterranean region, there is a culture of combining sweets with fresh fruit. French, Spanish, and Italian pastry chefs, bakers, and housewives are all fans of simple fruit cakes that highlight local produce.

Sweet Carrot and Cardamom Torte/
Torta di noci, carrote e cardamomo

I fell in love with the flavor combination of sweet carrots and cooling, herbal cardamom the first time I tasted them in a carrot-cardamom crème anglaise sauce. This flourless cake demonstrates the popular Medieval tradition of making vegetable–based desserts. Cardamom is believed to be an aphrodisiac in the Middle East, where it is added into coffees, teas, desserts, stocks, pilafs, and much more. Many of my friends laughed at me when I shared this with them, until February 2014, when WorldNews.com featured my Turkish Coffee with Cardamom recipe as part of their "Valentine's Aphrodisiac Snack" feature. Needless to say, my friends now believe me!

7 large eggs

1 cup plus 2 tablespoons (226 g) sugar, divided

1 teaspoon ground cardamom

¼ teaspoon unrefined sea salt or salt

1 teaspoon vanilla extract

Grated zest and juice of 1 orange

5 large carrots, peeled and grated (about 2½ cups, or 550 g)

1½ cups (120 g) finely ground walnuts

Yield: 10 servings

Heat the oven to 350°F (180°C). Coat a 10-inch (26 cm) springform pan with cooking spray.

Separate 5 of the eggs into yolks and whites. Set aside the whites. In the bowl of an electric mixer fitted with the paddle attachment, beat the 5 eggs yolks with the 2 remaining whole eggs. Add 1 cup (200 g) of the sugar, cardamom, salt, vanilla, and the orange zest and juice. Mix in the carrots and walnuts.

In a clean bowl and using a clean whisk attachment, use an electric mixer to beat the 5 egg whites to stiff peaks, adding the 2 tablespoons (26 g) of sugar once the whites are foamy. Gently fold the whites into the carrot batter.

Pour the batter into the prepared pan and bake for 50 minutes, or until a wooden skewer or cake tester inserted at the center of the cake comes out clean. Allow to cool for at least 1 hour before unmolding.

Mediterranean Tradition
Walnuts are native to many countries in the region. They are often crushed and added into sauces to top everything from chicken to vegetables and sweets. In southern Italy, Greece, Israel, and Turkey, they are often ground and used as flour in cakes such as this one. I often use them when creating gluten-free desserts for Passover.

Mediterranean Cooking Basics

Dried Beans

Purchasing dry beans and cooking them yourself is more economical and healthful than the canned variety. Common Mediterranean beans are cannellini, borlotti (cranberry), fava, chickpeas, pinto, broad, and black-eyed peas. They can all be prepared in advance and then stored in the refrigerator for up to 1 week for use in various recipes or tossed into salads, soups, and stews. All beans must be soaked overnight in cold water, or covered in boiling water for 1 hour prior to cooking. To prepare, drain the soaked beans and place them in a saucepan. Add 1 teaspoon salt, cover with water and bring to a boil over high heat. Reduce heat to medium-low, cover, and let cook until beans are tender, 25 to 50 minutes. (This could take longer depending on the size of the beans.) Drain and reserve the cooking water, which may come in handy to add to pasta.

Lentils

Unlike beans, lentils do not need to be soaked overnight. Instead, simply pour the lentils into a shallow bowl and sort through them with your fingers to make sure there are no stones or unwanted particles. Rinse in a colander, then add them directly to the recipe. To cook them on their own, cover with a double quantity of water or stock. Add salt, pepper, and a bay leaf. Bring to a boil over high heat, reduce heat to low and simmer, uncovered, until tender, about 25 minutes, depending on variety. (Red lentils are the quickest cooking, followed by green and brown, and then black.)

Polenta

Cornmeal is a staple all around the Mediterra nean region. To make polenta, bring 4 cups (950 ml) of water to a boil in a medium saucepan over high heat. Slowly pour in the cornmeal by the handful in a gentle stream, stirring or whisking simultaneously with a wooden spoon or whisk to avoid lumps, until the mixture starts to thicken, about 3 minutes.

Lower heat to medium-low (or a temperature that allows a very low simmer) and cook for at least 20 to 25 minutes, stirring about every 5 minutes. Be sure to crush any lumps that may form against the side of the pan. If the polenta is too thick, add ½ cup (120 ml) of water to soften it. Polenta is done when it easily comes away from the sides of the pan. Add salt and pepper to taste. Remove pan from heat and cool, allowing polenta to solidify.

Fresh Bread Crumbs

You'll be amazed at the difference switching from store-bought to fresh bread crumbs will make in your recipes. Begin with 1 dense, day-old, country–style loaf of bread. Cut the bread into 1-inch (2.5 cm) cubes and, working in batches if necessary, place them in a food processor, being careful not to fill it more than half way. Pulse on and off until the crumbs are as fine as possible. Freeze unneeded bread crumbs in a plastic freezer bag for up to 1 month.

Stocks

I highly recommend making your own stock because they taste better, are economical, and contain far less sodium than commercial varieties. Try making it in large quantities and freezing it in 1-quart (946 ml) portions so that it will always be on hand. Each of these recipes yields about 3½ quarts (14 cups or 3 L).

Vegetable Stock

1 onion, peeled and halved

1 carrot, peeled, trimmed, and halved

1 rib celery, trimmed and halved (can include leaves if desired)

4 ounces (115 g) cherry tomatoes

4 sprigs fresh basil with stems

1 small bunch fresh, flat-leaf parsley, with stems

½ teaspoon (5 g) unrefined sea salt or salt, plus more to taste

In a large stockpot, place the onion, carrot, celery, cherry tomatoes, basil, and parsley. Cover with 4 quarts (16 cups, or 4 L) cold water. Bring to a boil over high heat and reduce heat to medium-low. Add salt and simmer, uncovered, for 30 minutes. Drain stock and reserve. Discard the rest.

Seafood Stock

1 onion, peeled and halved

1 carrot, peeled, trimmed, and halved

1 rib celery, trimmed and halved

Shells from 2 pounds (910 g) shrimp

½ teaspoon unrefined sea salt or salt, plus more to taste

1 dried bay leaf

1 tablespoon whole black peppercorns

In a large stockpot, place the onion, carrot, celery, and shrimp shells. Cover with 4 quarts (16 cups, or 4 L) cold water. Bring to a boil over high heat and reduce heat to medium-low. Skim off the foam that floats to the top and discard. Add salt, bay leaf, and peppercorns. Simmer, uncovered, for 30 minutes. Drain stock and reserve. Discard the rest.

Chicken Stock

1 onion, peeled and halved

1 carrot, peeled, trimmed, and halved

1 rib celery, trimmed and halved

1¼ pounds (570 g) chicken bones or carcasses

1 teaspoon whole black peppercorns

5 green cardamom pods

½ teaspoon unrefined sea salt or salt

In a large stockpot, place the onion, carrot, celery, chicken bones, peppercorns, and cardamom. Cover with 4 quarts (16 cups, or 4 L) cold water. Bring to a boil over high heat and reduce heat to medium-low. Skim off the residue that forms on top of the stock and discard. Add salt and simmer, uncovered, for 40 minutes. Drain stock and reserve. Discard the rest.

Meat Stock

1 onion, peeled and halved

1 carrot, peeled, trimmed, and halved

1 rib celery, trimmed and halved

3 pounds (1.4 kg) beef, veal, lamb, or goat bones (shin, leg, rib, or collar), cut into 4-inch (10 cm) pieces

1 dried bay leaf

1 teaspoon whole black peppercorns

½ teaspoon unrefined sea salt or salt

In a large stockpot, place the onion (grilled or raw), carrot, celery, bones, bay leaf, and peppercorns. Cover with 4 quarts (16 cups, or 4 L) cold water. Bring to a boil over high heat and reduce heat to medium-low. Skim off the foam that floats to the top and discard. Add salt and simmer, uncovered, for 40 minutes. Drain stock and reserve. Discard the rest.

The Mediterranean Pantry

Due to the healthful nature of most Mediterranean ingredients, they can be purchased in many health food and organic markets as well as Mediterranean and Italian markets, and are increasingly available in most major supermarkets. In areas where there are large concentrations of people from countries in the region, Middle Eastern or European aisles can be found in supermarkets. If you need to substitute or omit an ingredient, don't feel bad! That's the way many delicious recipes have adapted over the centuries.

Aleppo Pepper: A traditional Turkish and Syrian burgundy colored variety of pepper named after the Syrian city on the Silk Road. The cuisine of the city of Aleppo, known as *Halaby* in Arabic, is considered to be one of the major cuisines of the Middle East. Substitute another mildly hot red pepper in recipes, if needed.

Baby Squid: Call your local market to make sure they have the smaller, tender squid in stock before making a trip.

Bulgur: Groats from various wheat species are parboiled, dried, and cracked into bits. Bulgur is available in fine, medium, and coarse varieties and is used in everything from sweets to snacks, salads, and main courses in Middle Eastern cuisine. Tabbouleh, kibbeh, and other items are made from it. Fine bulgur does not need to be cooked. It is simply covered in water and allowed to set for a few minutes until absorbed.

Candied Citron: Grown on a small, shrub-like tree, the large, yellow, oblong fruit with greenish pulp is found in Corsica, southern Italy, and the Greek islands. It is a popular addition to panettone, panforte, sweet breads, and cannoli filling. Although different, citrus zest is sometimes substituted.

Cavatelli: Little, cave-shaped pasta popular in the southern Italian regions of Basilicata, Calabria, and Puglia, where they are still made by hand. They are appreciated for their ability to absorb liquid.

Couscous: Eaten predominately in North Africa, Sicily, and the eastern Mediterranean, couscous is a tiny, round pasta made of semolina and coarsely ground durum wheat flour. The name originates from the Berber word *k'seksu*. Traditionally hand rolled, manufactured couscous is available in instant varieties in supermarkets. Israeli couscous, known as *moghrabieh* in Arabic, consists of larger, pearl-like pasta beads, and is a popular base for stews in the Levant.

Dried dates: Since fresh dates are not available in many places outside of North Africa and the Middle East, what the rest of the world refers to as a date, is actually a dried date. There are hundreds of varieties in the Middle East, but the ones that are consistently sweet, tender, and easy to find abroad are the Medjool. If the only dates you can find are extremely dry, soak them in citrus juice or water for a few hours until they plump up.

Dried figs: Popular throughout the region, Greece, the Italian region of Calabria, and Turkey export their high-quality products around the globe. Available in white and black varieties, it is the white that works best in the recipes in this book. As with dates, if the only figs you can find are extremely dry, soak them in citrus juice or water for a few hours until they plump up.

Dried sultanas (golden raisins): Golden raisins are a great addition to pilafs, cookies, breads, and puddings.

Expeller pressed canola oil: Whenever cooking with oils other than olive, search for "expeller pressed" on the label, which means that the oil was extracted without chemicals.

Feta cheese: A white, brine-cured cheese made in most Mediterranean countries. Its name is derived from the Greek word for "slice" and current EU regulations require that only feta produced in Greece uses its proper name. Feta from other countries is often sold as "white cheese." It is worth seeking out fresh, authentic varieties from Mediterranean markets, because their taste and temperature is very different from that found in supermarkets. Feta can be made from cow, goat, or sheep milk; it is sometimes made of a combination.

First cold-pressed, extra-virgin olive oil: Extracted from the first pressing of the olives, which denotes better quality and flavor. True extra-virgin olive oils are all first cold-pressed. Since many international consumers are not aware of this, many extra-virgin olive oils sold outside of "the Mediterranean" region will have both "Extra-Virgin" and the First Cold-Pressed marked on them.

Flax: A great source of omega-3, fiber, and lignans, flax was traditionally used for both medicinal and nutritive reasons. Nowadays, however, it is mostly health-conscious westerners who buy it to incorporate into smoothies, juices, baked goods, and shakes.

Greek yogurt: Greek and Greek-style yogurt is thicker, richer, and contains more protein than regular yogurt. I prefer the sheep/goat milk Greek yogurt that is sold in Mediterranean markets. Many other eastern Mediterranean countries also make delicious Greek-style yogurt. The Fage brand that is available in most supermarkets is made from cow's milk, and works well in all of the recipes in this book.

Green cardamom pods: Native to India, and considered to be India's favorite spice, cardamom is also the world's second most expensive spice. It is featured in everything from drinks to savory recipes and sweet desserts in the North African and Middle Eastern portions of the region. Cardamom can be bought whole in its pods, which need to be opened to remove its teeny black seeds, and ground or crushed in a mortar and pestle. Because the oils found in the seeds are extremely volatile, cardamom begins to lose its intoxicating aroma once ground.

Halloumi cheese: Made from cow's, goat's, and sheep's milk, or a combination of them, Halloumi is a semi-hard, unripened brined cheese from Cyprus, where it has been made using the same artisanal methods for millennia.

Harissa sauce: A fiery North African pepper paste that can be stirred into recipes or used as a condiment.

Maccheroni: A type of pasta ranging in shapes from those similar to rigatoni or the slightly more elongated *casareccio* style, often served with hearty tomato and meat sauces. This was traditionally a homemade shape that was synonymous to all pastas. The name is the origin for the English term *macaroni*.

Manchego: A Spanish hard, sheep's milk cheese made from milk of local Manchega breed of La Mancha sheep. Fresh Manchego is aged for only 2 weeks. "Cured" is typically aged for a minimum of 3 months and up to 6 months, while "aged" is aged for 1 year.

Medium-grain rice: Look for Calrose rice in organic stores or "Egyptian" rice in Mediterranean stores they contain quite a bit of starch and produce creamy recipes.

Medium-grain Spanish rice: La Bomba or Calasparra varieties are known for their ability to absorb liquid while retaining a slightly firm to the bite texture. They are often used in Paella recipes.

Orange blossom water: Water made from orange blossom oils and and is used as a flavoring for syrups and sweets.

Parmigiano-Reggiano: Aged cow's milk cheese from the Emilia-Romagna region of Italy. Italian law mandates that only Parmigiano-Reggiano made in specific areas can be called by its proper name. Look for "DOP" (protected designation of origin) varieties for the best quality.

Pecorino Romano: Aged sheep's milk cheese from the Lazio region of Italy around Rome. Pecorino denotes "coming from sheep," and many Italian locations have their own version. Pecorino Crotonese, Pecorino Sardo, Pecorino di Moliterno, and many others have their own distinct flavors and are worth sampling if you can find them.

Peeled fava beans: Used extensively in southern Italy, North Africa, and the Middle East, fava were one of the world's oldest crops. The peeled variety are dry, white, and require soaking before using.

Pickling salt: Similar to table salt, without the iodine, which causes vegetables to change color during the pickling process. It is often sold with canning materials.

Pomegranate molasses: Molasses made from pomegranate juice in the eastern Mediterranean. Used in dips, sauces, and as a garnish.

Preserved vine (grape) leaves: Since fresh vine leaves are only available for a short time, those preserved in brine are substituted when making stuffed vine leaves, or for wrapping and grilling fish and cheese.

Pure cinnamon: In the Mediterranean region, "pure" cinnamon is used. It has a more mellow flavor than the American variety which by law can be mixed with 20 percent Cassia. Look for true cinnamon, sometimes also called Sri Lankan cinnamon or Ceylon cinnamon.

Queso Cabrales: Northern Spanish semi-hard cheese made from pure, unpasteurized milk of cows, sheeps, or goats in the Asturias region. It is delicious on its own or blended into sauces.

Ras el Hanout: A Moroccan spice blend of up to twenty-seven spices that is increasingly available from major Western spice companies.

Red currants: Member of the gooseberry family native to Northern Europe, Spain, Italy, and Portugal. For recipes in this book, cranberries, raisins, or pomegranate seeds may be substituted.

Saffron: The world's most expensive spice is cultivated from the stigmas of the crocus flower in the autumn. Its English name is derived from the plural form of the feminine form of the Arabic word for yellow, *saffra*. Saffron provides a bright yellow pigment and unique flavor to drinks, savories, and sweets. Medicinally, saffron is said to increase energy, suppress coughs, have diuretic properties, rejuvenate the heart, and ease labor pains.

Tahini: A sesame seed paste referred to as *tahina* in Arabic that is used in baked goods, made into sweet halva, or used in a sauce for dipping pita, falafel, and crudités. This paste is also the base for hummus (whose real name is *Hummus bil Tahini* or Hummus with Tahini) and Baba Ghanoush.

Unfiltered extra-virgin olive oil: Refers to unfiltered olive oil that contains small particles of olive flesh, which reduces shelf life of the oil. Many people, myself included, feel that unfiltered olive oil has greater taste because the olive particles continue to flavor it. It can sometimes be found in chain supermarkets during holiday time.

Unrefined sea salt: This is my go-to salt. It is relatively inexpensive and has not been processed or been exposed to harsh chemicals. It contains a wide variety of minerals and elements necessary for optimal health, native to the area it comes from. It does not have added iodine, as does most commercial brands of table salt. Kosher salt, table salt, or other sea salts may be substituted in the recipes in this book.

White sesame: The attractive flowers of the tropical sesame plant produce sesame seeds as they dry up. They yield about 1 tablespoon (8 g) per pod. The seeds are also used to make culinary oils and paste.

Za'atar: A variety of thyme native to the Middle East. It can be used in breads, meat, poultry, soups, and stews. There is also a spice mix that includes wild thyme, which is referred to as za'atar in Arabic as well.

Bibliography

Books

Clark, Jacqueline and Farrow, Joanna. *Mediterranean; A Taste of the Sun in Over 150 Recipes*. London: Hermes House; 2001.

Davidson, Alan. *The Oxford Companion to Food*. New York: The Oxford University Press; 1999.

Diotaiuti, Luigi. *The Al Tiramisu Restaurant Cookbook: An Elevated Approach to Authentic Italian Cuisine*. Washington, DC: Create Space; 2013.

Ducasse, Alain and Dudemaine Sophie. *Ducasse Made Simple by Sophie*. USA: Worzalla; 2005.

Karyanis, Dean and Karyanis Catherine. *Regional Greek Cooking*. New York: Hippocrene Books; 2008.

Kaufman, Sheilah and Ilkin, Nur. *The Turkish Cookbook: Regional Recipes and Stories*. Boston: Interlink; 2010.

A Taste of Turkish Cuisine. New York: Hippocrene Books; 2002, 2013.

Sephardic Israeli Cuisine: A Mediterranean Mosaic. New York: Hippocrene Books; 2002.

Benkirane, Fettouma. La *Cuisine Marocaine*. France: Hachette Pratique.

Kostioukovitch, Elena: *Why Italians Love to Talk About Food*. New York: Farrar, Straus, and Giroux; 2006.

Mardam-Bey, Farouk. *Ziryab: Authentic Arab Cuisine*. Paris: Ici la Press; 2002.

Nasrallah, Nawal. *Delights from the Garden of Eden*. Connecticut: Equinox Publishing; 2003, 2013.

Riolo, Amy. *The Mediterranean Diabetes Cookbook*. Alexandria, VA: American Diabetes Association; 2011.

Arabian Delights: Recipes and Princely Entertaining Ideas from the Arabian Peninsula. Washington, DC: Capital Books; 2007.

Nile Style: Egyptian Cuisine and Culture. New York: Hippocrene Books; 2009, 2013.

Sitas, Amaranth. Kopiaste: *The Cookbook of Traditional Cyprus Food*. Cyprus: Kyriakou Ltd; 1983.

Wolfert, Paula. *The Food of Morocco*. New York: Harper Collins; 2011.

Yarasimos, Marianna. *500 Years of Ottoman Cuisine*. Istanbul: Boyut Publishing Group; 2007.

Zaouali, Lilia. *Medieval Cuisine of the Islamic World*. California: University of California Press; 2007.

Websites

Cleveland Clinic Wellness Editors. Top 5 Health Benefits of Going Mediterranean. 2012; Available at: www.clevelandclinicwellness.com/food/mediterranean-diet/Pages/top-5-health-benefits-of-going-mediterranean.aspx. Accessed March 1, 2014.

Diekman, Connie, Med, RD, LD, FADA, and Sotiropoulos, Sam. Beans, Nuts, and Seeds. Available at: www.netplaces.com/mediterranean-diet/focus-on-plant-based-foods/beans-nuts-and-seeds.htm. Accessed March 1, 2014.

Hauser, Annie. 7 Life-Enhancing Reasons to Eat Fish. 2014; Available at: www.everydayhealth.com/diet-nutrition/life-enhancing-reasons-to-eat-fish.aspx. Accessed on March 1, 2014.

Oldways Website. 50 Years of Nutrition Research. 2013; Available at: www.oldwayspt.org/resources/heritage-pyramids/mediterranean-diet-pyramid. Accessed January 25, 2014.

Olive Oil Source Editors. Enjoying Olive Oil. 1998–2014; Available at: www.oliveoilsource.com/page/enjoying-olive-oil. Accessed on January 25, 2014.

Portale Calabria Editors. 2010; Olio di Oliva di Calabria. PortaleCalabrria.com. Available at: www.portalecalabria.com/site/enogastronomia/olio/olio.asp. Accessed on January 25, 2014.

Riolo, Amy. 2012; Medieval Cuisine of Cyprus. Amyriolo.blogspot.com. Available at: www.amyriolo.blogspot.com/#!http://amyriolo.blogspot.com/2012/02/medieval-cuisine-of-cyprus.html. Accessed February 1, 2014.

Osborne, David K. The Mediterranean Diet: Greek Cuisine and Good Health. greekmedicine.net. 2007–2010; Available at: www.greekmedicine.net/therapies/The_Mediterranean_Diet.html. Accessed April 2, 2014.

Fruits and Veggies More Matters. Research: Fruits and Vegetables. Fruitsandveggiesmorematters.org 2008–2014. Available at: www.fruitsandveggiesmorematters.org/research. Accessed February 3, 2014.

Harlan, Timothy S., M.D. Why are Fruits and Nuts Good for You. Drgourmet.com. 2014; Available at: www.drgourmet.com/eatinghealthy/meddietfruitnuts.shtml. Accessed on February 3, 2014.

International Olive Council. Mediterranean Diet Pyramid. InternationalOliveOil.org. 2014; Available at: www.internationaloliveoil.org/estaticos/view/87-mediterranean-diet-pyramid. Accessed on April 2, 2014.

Patil, Kiran. Organic Facts. Organicfacts.net. 2014; Available at: www.organicfacts.net/health-benefits/vegetable/vegetables.html. Accessed on February 3, 2014.

Petruccelli, Raffaella, Mariotti, Pierluigi and Cerreti, Stefano. Olivo del Mediterraneo. www.pomologia.ivalsa.cnr.it. 2014; Available at: pomologia.ivalsa.cnr.it. Accessed on February 3, 2014.

Toback, Rebecca. 22 Mediterranean Diet Recipes. Health.com. 2014; Available at: www.health.com/health/gallery/0,20718485,00.html. Accessed on April 15, 2014.

Tri-Lamb Group. Lamb and Your Health. LeanonLamb.com. 2011; Available at: www.leanonlamb.com/nutrition/. Accessed on April 15 2014.

Magazine/Newspaper Articles

Food and Recipe Network. Healthy Mediterranean Recipes and Menus. EatingWell.com. 2014. Available at: www.eatingwell.com/recipes_menus/collections/healthy_mediterranean_recipes. Accessed on February 3, 2014.

Hiatt, Kurtis. Mediterranean Diet. Health.USNews.com. 2013; Available at: health.usnews.com/best-diet/mediterranean-diet/recipes. Accessed May 9, 2014.

Kolata, Gina. "Mediterranean Diet Shown to Ward off Heart Attack and Stroke," the New York Times. February 25, 2013.

Terranova, Giovanna. La qualità dell'olio per curare i tumori scoperti all'Unical i benefici dell'extravergine. Ilquotidianodellacalabria.it. May 18, 2014; Available at: www.ilquotidianodellacalabria.it/news/idee-societa/721861/La-qualita-dell-olio-per-curare.html. Accessed May 19, 2014.

Journals

Allison, Aubrey. NPR: The Salt. For the Mind and Body. Study Finds Mediterranean Diet Boosts Both. November 5, 2013; Available at: www.npr.org/blogs/thesalt/2013/11/05/242994376/for-mind-body-study-finds-mediterranean-diet-boosts-both. Accessed January 10, 2014.

Environmental Defense Fund. EDF Seafood Selecter. The Benefits of Eating Fish. Available at: seafood.edf.org/benefits-eating-fish. Accessed April 10, 2014.

Godman, Heidi. Harvard Health Publications. Adopt a Better Diet Now for Better Health Later. 2013; Available at: www.health.harvard.edu/blog/adopt-a-mediterranean-diet-now-for-better-health-later-201311066846. Accessed March 1, 2014.

Harvard Health Publications. The Mediterranean Diet. HelpGuide.org. 2013; Available at: www.helpguide.org/life/mediterranean-diet.htm. Accessed May 9, 2014.

Huffington Post Staff. Mediterranean Diet May Protect Against Diabetes Study Suggests. August 20, 2013; Available at: www.huffingtonpost.com/2013/08/20/mediterranean-diet-diabetes-type-2_n_3770063.html. Accessed January 3, 2014.

Johnson, Kathy. 10 Commandments of the Real Mediterranean Diet. ABC.net.au. 2013; Available at: www.abc.net.au/health/thepulse/stories/2013/04/15/3737114.htm. Accessed May 10, 2014.

Mayo Clinic Staff. Mediterranean Diet a Hearth Healthy Eating Plan. MayoClinic.org. 1998–2014; Available at: www.mayoclinic.com/health/mediterranean-diet/CL00011. Accessed May 10, 2014.

Omega-3 In Fish: How Eating Fish Helps Your Heart. MayoClinic.org. 1998–2014. Available at: www.mayoclinic.org/diseases-conditions/heart-disease/in-depth/omega-3/art-20045614. Accessed May 10, 2014.

Nauert, Rick, Ph.D. Mediterranean Diet May Benefit Mind as well as Body. PsychCentral.com. 2014; Available at: www.psychcentral.com/news/2013/09/04/mediterranean-diet-may-benefit-mind-as-well-as-body/59177.html. Accessed May 19, 2014.

Preidt, Robert. Chocolate, Tea, Berries May Cut Diabetes Risk. HealthDay.com. 2014; Available at: consumer.healthday.com/diabetes-information-10/misc-diabetes-news-181/choco-tea-berries-diabetes-j-of-nutrition-u-east-anglia-release-batch-1107-684032.html. Accessed March 4, 2014.

Reuters. Mediterranean Diet's Anti-Diabetes Benefits Revealed. CBSNews.com. January 7, 2014; Available at: www.cbsnews.com/news/mediterranean-diets-anti-diabetes-benefits-revealed/. Accessed March 4, 2014.

Seafood Health Facts. Seafood and Nutrition. Seafood & Current Dietary Recommendations. Available at: www.seafoodhealthfacts.org/seafood_nutrition/practitioners/seafood_dietary.php. Accessed April 10, 2014.

Thomas, Mathew. Lyme Disease and the Mediterranean Diet: A Review of Literature. Mathewgthomas.weebly.com. 2012; Available at: www.matthewgthomas.weebly.com/uploads/2/4/4/6/24464532/lyme_disease__med_diet-_a_review_of_literature-final.pdf. Accessed March 4, 2014.

University of Exeter. Mediterranean Diet is Good for the Mind, Research Confirms. Science Daily, September 3, 2013; Available at: www.sciencedaily.com/releases/2013/09/130903101951.htm.

Index

Acknowledgments

I have destiny to thank for enabling me to get to know so many people and places in the Mediterranean region and at such an intimate level. I believe that it truly "takes a village" to make a good chef—and in my case, that village is a global one. I am honored and proud to say that I have learned from amazing cooks in places that I never dreamed I would even visit. For all of you who have shared a kitchen or a meal with me, I thank you.

My nonna, Angela Magnone Foti, taught me to cook and bake, as well as valuable lessons that served me outside of the kitchen. She gave me my first cookbook and showed me how cooking was not a mundane chore, but a form of magic that could unite people across distances and time. I owe my career to her, and would give anything to be able to share more time with her. My Yia Yia, Mary Michos Riolo, shared her beloved Greek traditions with me, and I am happy to say that they have become woven into my culinary fabric as well. My earliest memories of cooking were with my mother, Faith Riolo, who would sit me on the counter and roll more meatballs and cookies than I could count. She taught me that food was not just something we eat to nourish ourselves, but an edible gift that could be given to express love. I owe my love of food history and anthropology to my father, Rick Riolo, for planting the desire to answer the question, "I wonder how they eat . . ?" in my mind since childhood. It's a type of culinary curiosity that is never completely satisfied and gives me the motivation to continue my work each day.

I would probably never have published a cookbook if it weren't for my mentor, Sheilah Kaufman, who patiently taught me much more than I ever planned on learning. To my dear friend Rosa Vilella, may your memory live on through the recipes that you shared with everyone you knew. I am very thankful to my partner, Chef Luigi Diotaiuti, for being a continuous source of inspiration and motivation, and for enabling me to share my passions and philosophies.

In Italy, I thank my cousin Angela Riolo for sharing my passion and continuously supplying me with authentic Calabrian recipes. In Rome, I thank Liana Mari, Mauro Lesti, and Marialuisa DiMatteo for your continued support. I also thank Luigi and Maria Fabbiano for sharing so much with me over the years.

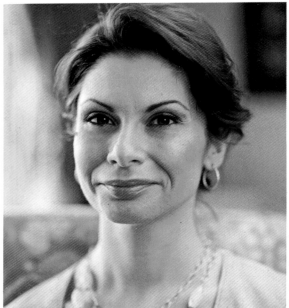

Michael Stewart Photography

In Egypt, I am forever indebted to Dr. Amira Mohsen for her patience and assistance in helping me conduct my research, and to Soad El Tanbedawy for sharing so many of her recipes with me. To my family in Luxor, the Edris family—Ahmed, Mohamed, Mahmoud, Omaima, and Koty, Mahmoud Fathy el Kady, Gerges Samwell, Ahmed Nouby Moussa, Chef Tarek Mohamed, Chef Ahmed Hashem, Chef Heggag, and Chef Hussein— thank you for your help and support.

Thank you to Dr. Norton Fishman, Kathleen Ammalee Rogers, Dr. Beth Tedesco, and Dr. Mary Lee Esty for enabling me to overcome my illness and fulfill my dreams. To my dear friend Susan Simonet, you are the sister I never had. I truly appreciate the positive endorsements of Lidia Bastianich, Chef Jason Roberts, Dr. John Principe, and Chef Luigi Diotaiuti. It is a pleasure working with all of you.

I would like to thank my editor, Jill Alexander, Betsy Gammons, and Anne Re for assisting me with the creation of this book. A huge thank you to Dr. John Principe and Dr. Martha Kern for sharing their knowledge and insight. I would also like to thank every shopkeeper, housewife, taxi driver, chef, fisherman, farmer, and restaurateur who took the time to discuss food with me and provided me with additional insight.